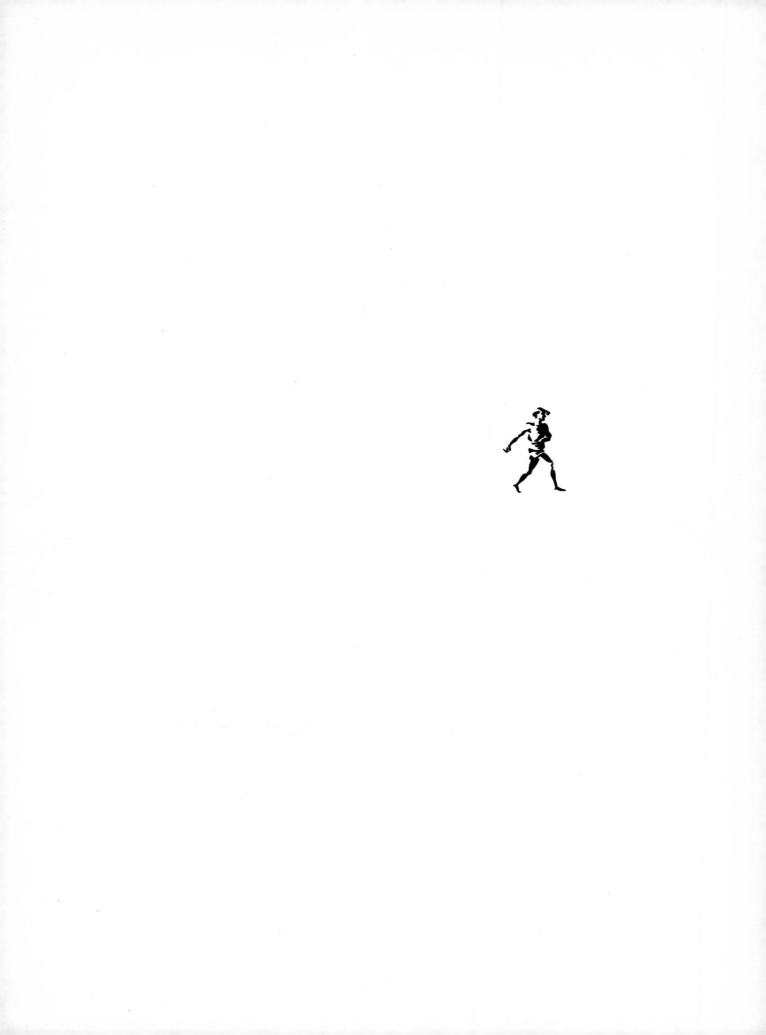

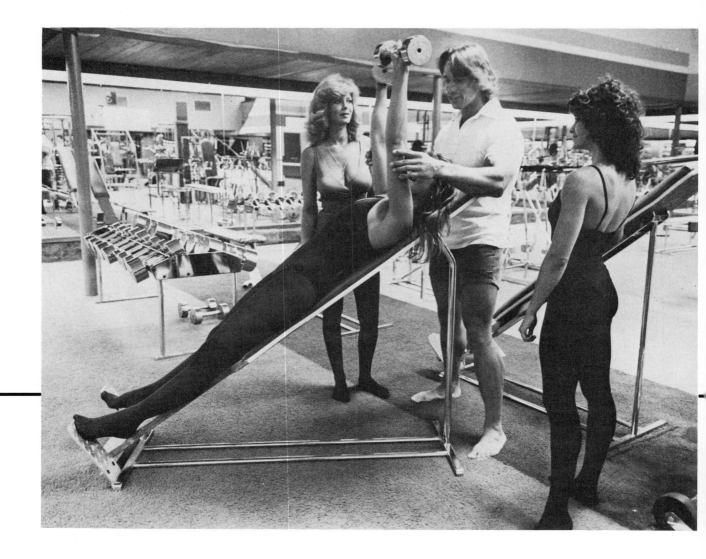

Also by Arnold Schwarzenegger

Arnold: The Education of a Bodybuilder
with Douglas Kent Hall

Also by Douglas Kent Hall

On the Way to the Sky
The Superstars
Let 'er Buck!
Rock & Roll Retreat Blues
Rodeo
Van People: The Great American Rainbow Boogie
The Master of Oakwindsor

Arnold's Bodyshaping for Women

by
Arnold Schwarzenegger

with Douglas Kent Hall

Simon and Schuster • New York

Published by Simon and Schuster
A Division of Gulf & Western Corporation
Simon & Schuster Building
Rockefeller Center
1230 Avenue of the Americas
New York, New York 10020
SIMON AND SCHUSTER and colophon are
trademarks of Simon & Schuster

Photographs by Douglas Kent Hall
Illustrations by Paula Joseph

Designed by Libra Graphics, Inc.
Manufactured in the United States of America

   6 7 8 9 10 11 12 13

Library of Congress Cataloging in Publication Data

Schwarzenegger, Arnold
   Arnold's bodyshaping for women.

   1. Weight lifting. 2. Exercise for women.
3. Women—Nutrition. I. Hall, Douglas Kent,
joint author. II. Title.
GV546.S38   613.7′045   79-17911

ISBN 0-671-24301-2

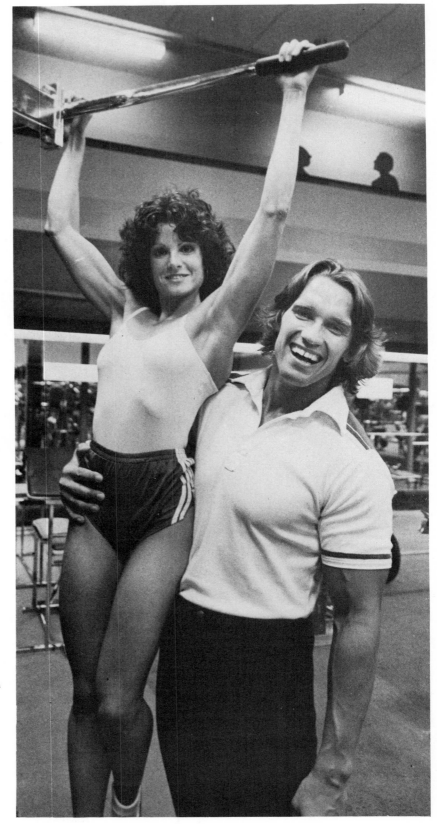

TO MY MOTHER

And to those people who pioneered weight training for women and whose dedication and determination have inspired millions of women to make weight training a way to a healthier life. In the forefront are Virginia Smith, Betty Weider, Lucia Zurkowski, Joyce Grau, and Dot Kawashima and The American Association of Physical Fitness Centers and its employees.

A special thanks to Rudy and Virginia Smith, Roy and Lucia Zurkowski, Betty and Joe Weider, Joyce Grau and Lisa Lyon for their help on this book.

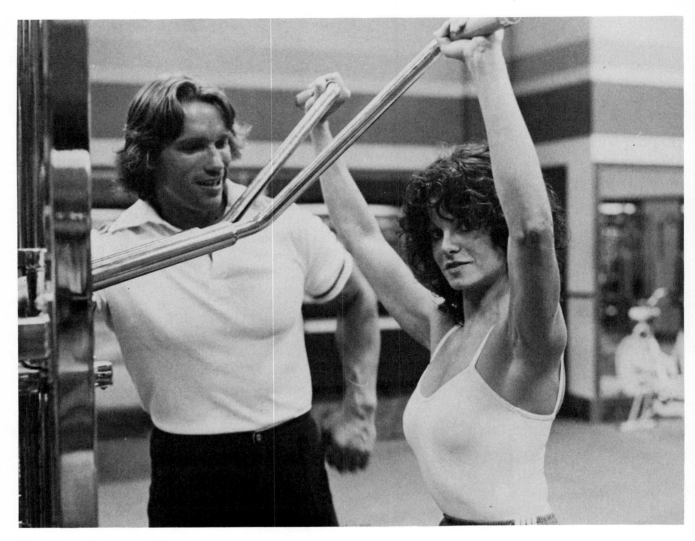

Here I am having another great workout with Lisa Lyon, who is the women's world champion in bodybuilding.

O F THE MANY WAYS to exercise your body, resistance training is the most complete and direct. Running and jogging will train your legs and cardiovascular system and help you release negative tension and frustration. Swimming is great for flexibility and stretching the muscles. Tennis, squash, skiing, and many other sports work selected areas of the body and promote coordination. Yoga is valuable for gaining control over muscles by bringing together mind and body. But resistance training, which achieves all of the above, has the additional advantage of isolating and working specific muscles in every area of the body, making it the most economical way to achieve the greatest results in the shortest amount of time.

The principle behind resistance training is very simple. If you lift your forearm, your biceps muscle (the muscle in the front of your upper arm) must work to overcome the resistance created by the weight of your forearm and hand. If you then add more weight to your hand—a book, a hammer, a dumbbell—the biceps must work harder to overcome the increased resistance and lift it. When you work a muscle, blood rushes in to supply it with nutrients and take away waste materials. The harder the muscle works, overcoming increased resistance, the more energy it needs to keep going. The energy supply in the bloodstream comes from the food you eat and from the excess stores you have put aside in the form of fat. Therefore, if you do not increase the amount of food you take in and work your muscles harder, you automatically begin to use up the fat in the vicinity of the muscle you are training. Further, if you cut down on the amount you eat and work the muscles harder, you will burn up fat even faster.

There are both positive and negative resistance. When you lift your forearm, you are overcoming positive resistance. If you let your arm back down slowly, you create negative resistance. You should understand that your muscle benefits as much from negative as from positive resistance. By making use of both in workouts, you save time and increase the effectiveness of the workout.

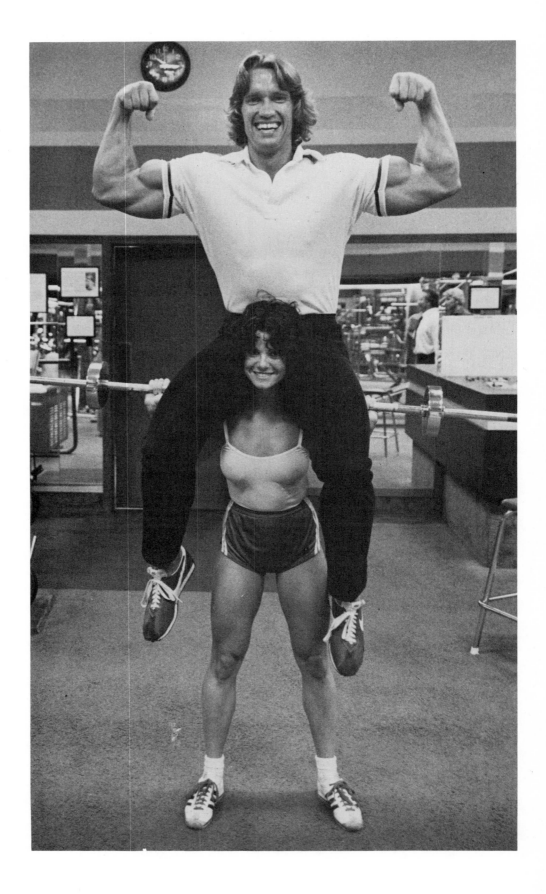

Titles Won

1965	Jr. Mr. Europe (Germany)
1966	Best Built Man of Europe (Germany)
1966	Mr. Europe (Germany)
1966	International Powerlifting Championship (Germany)
1967	NABBA Mr. Universe, amateur (London)
1968	NABBA Mr. Universe, professional (London)
1968	German Powerlifting Championship
1968	IFBB Mr. International (Mexico)
1969	IFBB Mr. Universe, amateur (New York)
1969	NABBA Mr. Universe, professional (London)
1970	NABBA Mr. Universe, professional (London)
1970	Mr. World (Columbus, Ohio)
1970	IFBB Mr. Olympia (New York)
1971	IFBB Mr. Olympia (Paris)
1972	IFBB Mr. Olympia (Essen, Germany)
1973	IFBB Mr. Olympia (New York)
1974	IFBB Mr. Olympia (New York)
1975	IFBB Mr. Olympia (Pretoria, South Africa)

Contents

WOMEN AND EXERCISE

THE EXERCISE SERIES

Women and Exercise

Women and Fitness

When I started competing in Europe, a woman's beauty contest was always held in connection with the men's competition. These women looked fantastic. Almost all of them were on physical fitness programs, working with weights and doing other kinds of training. As I traveled, competing and giving bodybuilding exhibitions, I saw in most of the big cities of England, Holland, France, and Germany progressive gymnasiums which were either coed or had separate facilities for women.

At first, it surprised me to see women training with weights. They weren't just doing passive exercises with vibrator belts and roller massagers; they were actually working out, doing bench presses, presses behind the neck, squats, leg extensions, cable pulls—in fact, almost everything I did myself. I realized that these women, the most beautiful in Europe, had great bodies because they had used weights to reshape and bring their bodies to as near a perfect state as they could. What surprised me most was that working with weights had not made them look at all muscular. Instead, resistance training—training with weights —only seemed to emphasize all of their feminine attributes, leaving them more beautiful, curvacious, and appealing.

I took it for granted that women in America participated in similar exercise programs. But when I came to the United States, I found this wasn't true. Here, it seemed, women still treated themselves as weaker, inferior individuals; they went to cream-puff gyms (called spas) and did

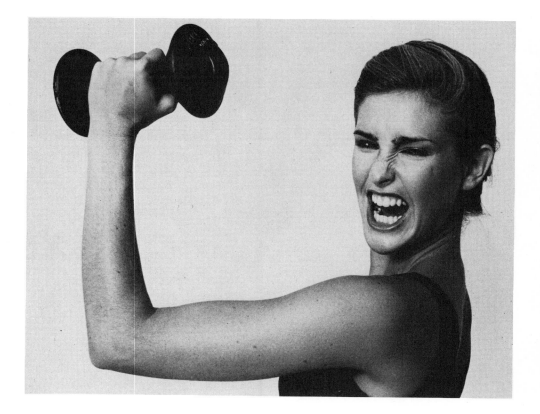

some very passive exercises. They would hang on to vibrator belts, talk to their neighbor for 5 or 10 minutes, sit in a Jacuzzi, take a shower, end with a rubdown, and that constituted their workout!

In fact, I distinctly remember a sign I saw in a gym in California: A HORSE SHOULD SWEAT, A MAN SHOULD PERSPIRE, BUT A WOMAN SHOULD ONLY GLISTEN.

I also remember that shortly after I arrived in California, a woman asked me what she could do to take the flab off her triceps (the muscles at the back of the upper arm). I suggested an exercise that called for a pair of light dumbbells. She freaked out!

Fortunately, that attitude is changing. I think it had a lot to do with the women's liberation movement. As the idea of sexual equality gained more acceptance, women started to believe in the philosophy of equality in everything. Getting away from the fallacy of feminine weakness and getting into shape physically was part of it.

A few years ago when I became a member of the Association of Physical Fitness Centers, women were saying they were tired of being shoved off in a corner and merely tolerated. They wanted the same size gyms men had, with more sophisticated equipment that would allow them to train harder. Women told gym owners they needed a better selection of weights; they wanted less emphasis on vibrating belts and other equipment that did almost nothing for their bodies. They wanted resistance machines, cable machines, weight racks, and benches.

That was the beginning of the big change in America for women and fitness. Many women's gymnasiums are now as well equipped as men's gyms, and the improvements are continuing rapidly due to the efforts of the Association of Physical Fitness Centers. Women are being given the opportunity to do as they like without fear of adverse criticism. Women are using heavier weights *with only favorable results.* Women are in tough competition against men in tennis, skiing, and other sports. Women are proving that they are indeed equal to men—not only mentally, but also physically—and are beginning to live up to their physical potential.

The Weaker Sex

The statement that women are the weaker sex is as unfair as it is ridiculous. In terms of sheer force, it is safe to say that men, with their larger bone structure and greater muscle mass, are potentially stronger. But in endurance, women excel. Their bodies are prepared for a feat of endurance unknown to men: pregnancy and the bearing of children.

During my youth in Austria, I used to swim and keep up with all the championships. I noticed that most of the records in long distance swimming, such as swimming the English Channel, were made or broken by women. In everyday life, too, women can sustain physical stress for longer periods of time than men. This became very clear to me after I had won my first Mr. Universe title and gone home to Austria for a visit. One of my relatives had a new baby, a few months old. She handed the baby to me to hold. I held her gently because I didn't want to hurt her. I was nervous because I didn't *think* I could hold the baby the right way. I cradled her with one arm, and supported her with the other arm. After a few minutes, this baby started feeling heavier and heavier. I could feel her weight in my shoulders and my arms. Finally, I said, "She's a nice baby—beautiful. Here, you can have her back. I don't want to drop her." Then I watched my cousin carry her baby almost continuously for the rest of the day. She never once mentioned that her arms were getting tired.

The average woman could not work out with the amount of weight I handle easily every day. She could probably try all her life and never come close to doing it. But she could very well build herself up to the point of doing as many or more repetitions with a lighter weight. She could possibly out-distance me on the track. And she is certainly capable of out-swimming me (that extra layer of fatty tissue between the skin and muscles that makes a woman rounder also adds buoyancy and insulation against the prolonged shock of being in cold water).

Women and Weights

The biggest change in women in the past few years—the one that has probably brought about the most progress—has been in their attitude. I see it happening in the reactions female reporters have to bodybuilding when they interview me for TV, magazines, radio, and newspapers, and in the frequency with which women come to me for advice about exercise.

At parties, I hear so many problems in one evening, I feel almost like a doctor doing hospital rounds. It usually begins with one woman and a question like, "Can women improve their thighs with weight training?" My answer is, "Yes, absolutely. You can tone up the muscles in your legs and improve the contours of your legs." By that time, five or ten other women are waiting, each with a question to ask.

"I have a problem in my lower back. I can't play tennis."

And another says, "I have such bony shoulders I'm embarrassed to wear a strapless dress. What can I do?"

"I have no calves."

"My ankles are too thick."

Sooner or later, I begin making appointments for the next day— for private sessions at the gym. But there is never enough time for me to follow through, and I haven't found a book I can recommend that really gives women a comprehensive training program. There are numerous books on remaking yourself with artificial things—makeup, clothing, hair

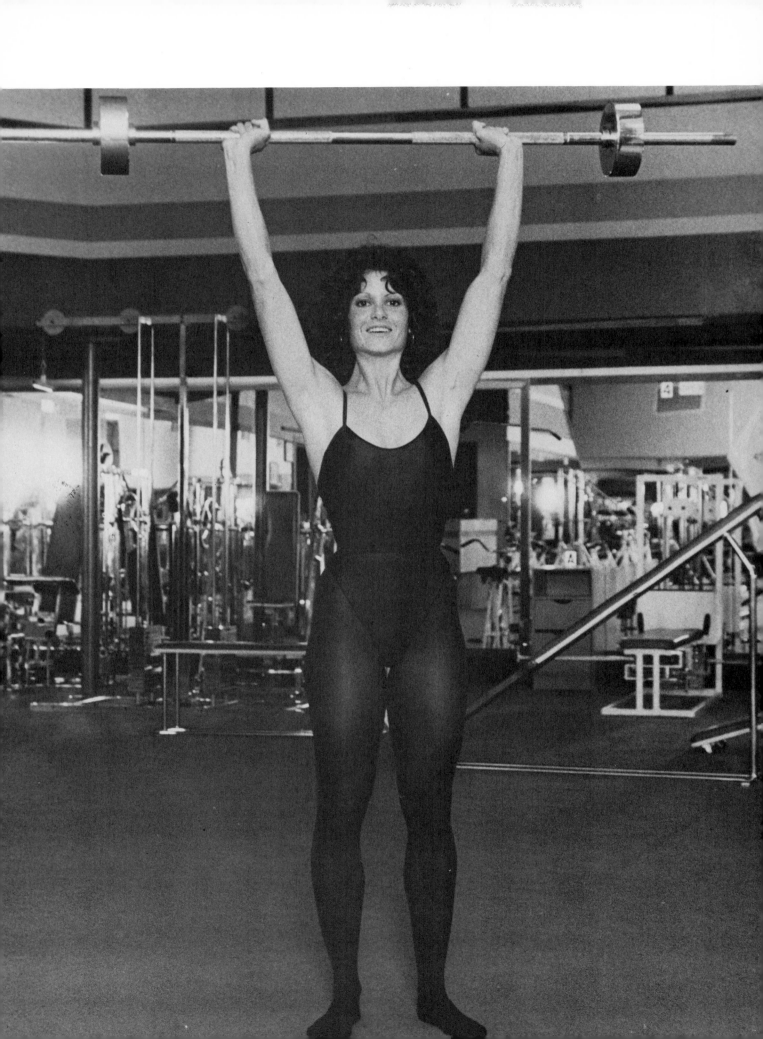

styles—but nothing, in my opinion, that deals comprehensively with the *real* physical you—with your body.

I finally suggested that these women come to the seminars I was holding for men. And eventually I began conducting seminars exclusively for women. The women attending these seminars were seriously interested in training with weights, of course, but they were always skeptical. They wanted to work out, but they didn't want the same results from working with weights that men got. I explained that unless she has a hormone imbalance—which is rather rare and, once discovered, can usually be corrected—a woman cannot develop the same kind of muscles a man can build through exercise. The main reason is chemical and genetic. A normal woman has more estrogen (the female hormone) and less testosterone (the male hormone) than a man.

Up to the time of puberty, the differences between the bodies of boys and girls are relatively few. By playing the same games and doing the same things boys do, girls often grow and develop similarly to the ways boys do. For this reason, they're sometimes called tomboys. Then at puberty, testosterone from the testes is introduced into the bloodstream of boys. They develop longer bones, more muscle mass, and the potential for greater body weight. At the same time—though puberty usually occurs somewhat earlier in girls—estrogen from the ovaries flows into the bloodstream of girls to influence the changes that are peculiar to the feminine body: the slightly thicker layer of fat between the skin and muscle tissue (a woman's body contains approximately 25 percent more fat cells than a man's, meaning she also has fewer muscle cells) and the

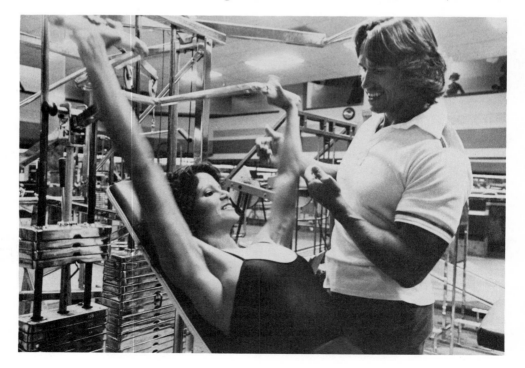

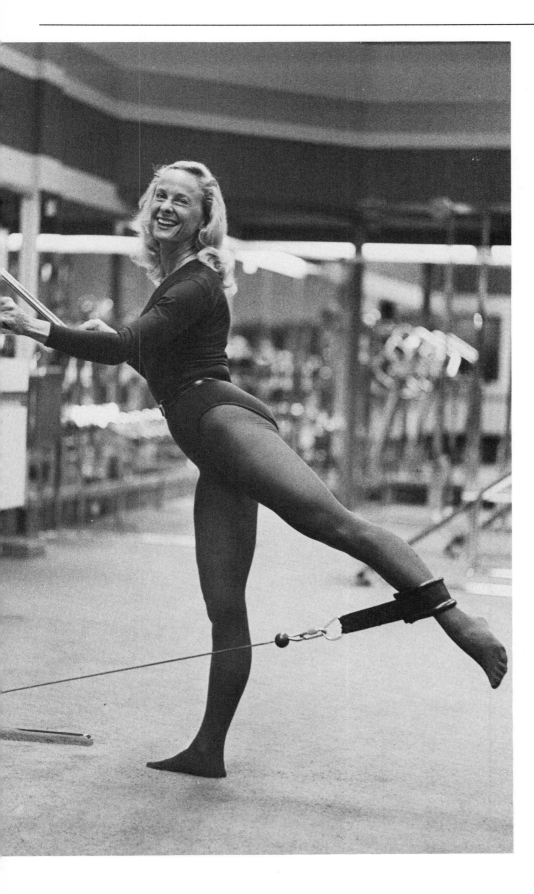

Virginia Smith, a grandmother and also the director of women's activities for one of the largest health club chains, has been working out with weights for twenty-five years.

structural differences that prepare a woman's body for childbearing (wider hips, the somewhat different angle at which the thigh bone inserts into the hip sockets, etc.). The first—that extra number of fat cells—gives a woman her more curvacious body. The second influences a woman's walk and carriage and is also one reason women often need to pay special attention when exercising thighs, knees, and lower back. Vigorous exercise serves only to emphasize the kind of body—male or female—we already have, the body nature has given us. Generally speaking, a man will become more angular and muscular, and a woman more curvacious with softer-looking lines. Most convincing are the women I could point to who have worked out for years in a gym. They are fit, well proportioned, beautiful, sexy, and *not* muscular looking.

Cellulite

To your body, fat is fat. You may call it cellulite or any other name if you wish, but the truth is your body handles all fat in the same manner. It goes through the liver, a certain amount is taken out and used in the process of maintaining normal body functioning, and the excess is stored in your body—especially in those neglected areas where the muscles have gone unused for years. Sometimes this fat collects in unsightly, sagging pockets along the thighs, the backs of the arms and in apronlike accumulations in the lower abdomen. Because of its cellular appearance —like a bunch of ping-pong balls trapped under the skin—it's called cellulite. To me, this condition merely indicates two things: a person badly out of shape and/or overweight.

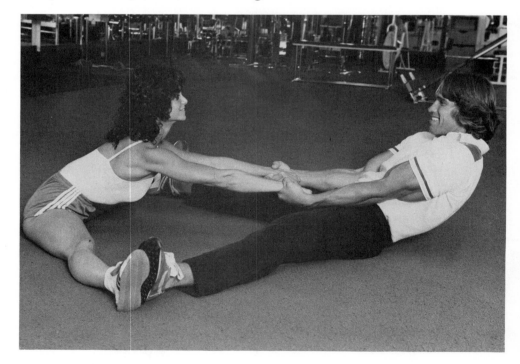

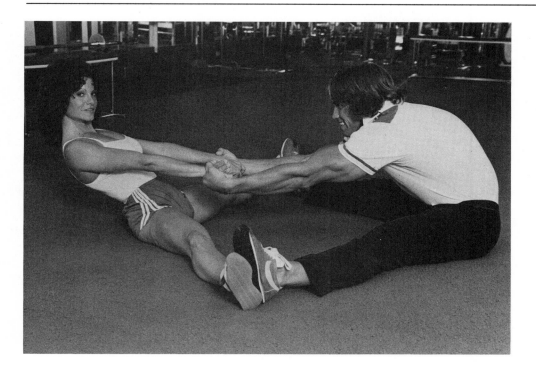

Fat can be eliminated by a combination of two things: first, by limiting and balancing your diet to cut down your intake of fats and to provide the extra protein and other nutrients necessary to rebuild the lean muscle tissue you need to smooth out the problem areas; and, second, by following a program of exercises designed to strengthen and tone the unused muscles in those areas where fat accumulated in the first place. Cellulite may be the last fat to go, but eventually it will. It took time for your muscles to weaken and diminish and for this excess fat to pile up, and it will take time and effort to bring these areas back to a smoother, more pleasing state.

Let me add a word of caution about the so-called special secrets for losing cellulite, such as deep, abusive massage, injections, surgery. None of these is really effective. In some cases, in fact, these remedies have been proven to be extremely harmful.

The Bust

"Arnold, what can I do to increase my bust size?" I hear the same question in every seminar, and my answer is always the same: In most instances, no exercises can really change the size of your breasts. This can only be accomplished by injections or surgery—neither of which I recommend. Exercise, however, can *improve* the look of your bust and perhaps make it *appear* to have increased in size.

What will happen is this: Certain of the exercises I suggest will expand your ribcage; other exercises will develop, firm up, and build the pectoral muscles that lie under and support your breasts. The breasts themselves are made up of glands, fatty tissue, and connecting ligaments and are not likely to change very much. However, as a result of the increased efficiency of your blood transport system and what that does to tone up all the glands and organs, the breasts may be affected slightly

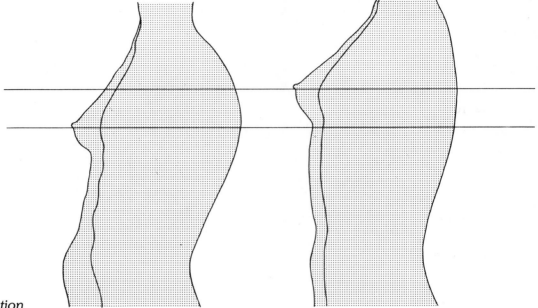

By developing the pectorals, the foundation muscles underlying the breast, you can increase your bust measurement.

—this could be especially true for teenage girls still in the process of developing—but normally, there is *no* detectable change in size. Your A or D cup will likely remain just that.

On the other hand, due to the development and toning of the pectoral muscles, the muscles in the back, and a slight expansion of the ribcage, you may go from a 34A or D to a 36A or D; and with the improvement in posture, your bustline will look and feel better.

Being In Shape

I was invited, one weekend after the Robert Kennedy Celebrity Tennis Tournament, to spend a few days with the Shriver family in Hyannisport, Massachusetts. I had been impressed with the Kennedys for years before I got to know them, because of their political achievements and the charitable work they have done. What made me admire them even more was that they were all—whether male or female, young or old—involved in physical activities.

I went up to Hyannisport to spend what I thought would be a slow, relaxing weekend, but I never in my life played so many different sports. I believe I found out the reason various members of the family achieve as much as they do. They work hard to keep themselves in great physical shape, which gives them abundant energy and stamina for their political and intellectual pursuits. They get out early in the morning and play till late at night, sailing in the early morning, water skiing later, playing football, volleyball, basketball, soccer, and tennis in the afternoon. When most other people are wiped out and go to sleep, they're still either working or playing. They try to use 100 percent of their potential. And that's not something I can say about many people I know. Everyone in the family participated. It seemed to make no difference at all whether they were men or women.

The real surprise came in the afternoon when, after what had already seemed a long, full day, Bobby Shriver said, "Let's go to the gym." During the hour we spent working out with weights, I discovered he has been enthusiastic about resistance training for years. For him, it is not only a matter of staying in shape; it is also a way of relaxing and loosening up.

When we got back to the house, there was just time to dress for a dinner party. I was seated next to Eunice Shriver. She asked me what she could do to get in shape. I thought she was joking. But she really wanted to know. She was interested in firming up certain areas of her body she felt she had neglected. I showed her a few exercises she could do at home (which are among the exercises discussed later in this book). When I finished, she and Ethel Kennedy said we should put together an exercise program for Rose Kennedy, who is in her eighties. They were serious; they had no intention of figuring out ways to make Rose less active. They said that although she already spends 1½ or 2 hours walking, Rose herself was interested in finding a program to help keep herself firm, limber, and in good shape.

None of us gets enough of the right kind of exercise. And in most instances, women are going to get less exercise on a 9-to-5 job than they would if they stayed home and did an average amount of housework. Driving to the office, getting out of the car, walking to the elevator, going from the elevator to an office, and then sitting at a desk for the next 8 hours is hardly enough exercise to maintain a healthy body.

Facing the Modern World

As you become more competitive with men, you must be ready to meet many of the same problems men have. You will have to prepare yourself not only for the rigors of your new life, with its new schedules and burdens, but also for the pressures you'll come under in the complex worlds of business, industry, and government.

Ten or twenty years ago, men bore the burden of most of this pressure, and it showed up very clearly in the statistics about heart attacks. For every seven men who had a heart attack, there was only one woman who had a heart attack. Now, however, the numbers are gradually moving toward a balance, which shows that heart disease is not really sex related (aside from the fact that women are thought to be protected by estrogen in early adulthood).

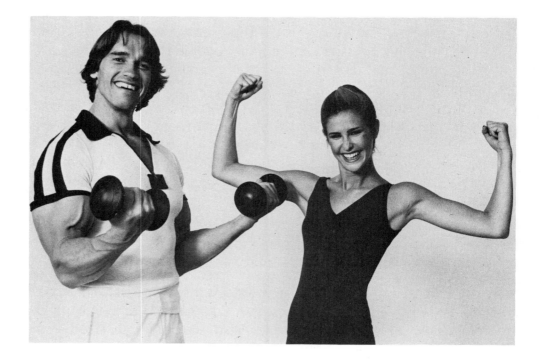

As a woman living in a new and changing age, you should know that being in shape makes sense. You will be more alert and experience an overall increase in mental energy. You will be even tempered and less likely to become impatient. You will avoid frustration which may be detrimental to your job and may actually impair your ability to function in a highly competitive world.

Being in shape also means looking good. When men go to a bar, to the beach, or to a party, what do they look for in a woman? They don't give every woman they see an intelligence test. They don't spend an hour to see if she gives off the right vibrations. Right or wrong, men and women begin by putting you, me, everyone, through a visual test. This probably happens in 90 percent of our social situations. That first visual impression is what creates an initial interest. If you weigh 200 pounds or look out of shape; if you don't take care of yourself, your hair, fingernails, and face, you'll probably be passed over.

People want to be aesthetically satisfied visually—whether they are looking at a body, a building, or a car. That's why packaging plays such an important part in commerce. People don't choose things for their functional qualities nearly as often as for their looks. Design is important in our lives. When a company decides to erect a new building, the first thing it does is hire architects and designers to plan both a pleasing interior and exterior. Why? Because they know people's initial impressions are formed by appearance.

Let's say you weigh 150 pounds (30 pounds overweight), and you wear a dress three sizes larger than you did a few years ago. You don't like being this way, but you haven't done anything to change it. You may use makeup that gives your face a hollow look, or style your hair in a way that makes your face slender, or buy dark-colored dresses in loose, blousy shapes that minimize the proportions of your body, and wear heels high enough to trim your ankles and give your legs a longer look. Does any of this sound familiar? Maybe it's all right as long as you can stay covered up. But it's not healthy and it won't work all the time. Instead of concentrating on artificial solutions to hide your problems, take steps to eliminate them—forever.

Sometimes the problem is not one of overweight. You can be out of shape at any weight. Four years ago, I had dinner with a woman named Lisa. She was so thin and fragile that if I had said something very strong, she would have fallen apart. She was too fragile—inside and out—for me and I soon forgot her. Recently, I accidentally ran into her in a shoe store. She was standing at the counter in shorts. I didn't recognize her at first. All I saw was this woman with a great body. She had unbelievable legs, fantastic calves, a small waist, and nice breasts. She was really striking—the kind of woman you stop to look at. Finally, when she

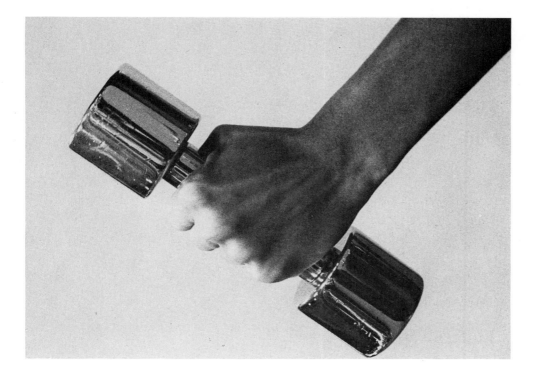

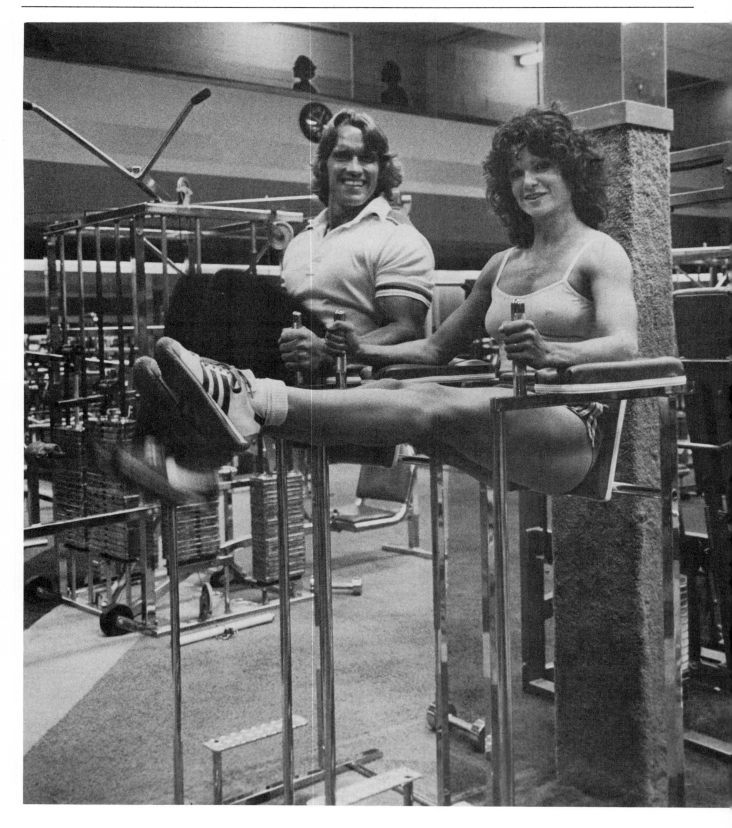

turned to leave, I realized it was Lisa. The change was incredible. I asked what she was doing there. She said she was buying new running shoes, her fourth pair—she had already worn out three pairs. I told her she looked great, that I couldn't believe she was the same person. "Thank you," she said. "I've been running. But mainly, I've been training with weights." She began talking about deadlifts, about bench presses. I was amazed.

I invited her to the gym the next day. We worked out together, doing some incredible things. Training had had anything but adverse effects. She had developed a very shapely, stunning body—a knockout. More than that, she had totally changed her attitude about herself. Looking at her, I felt as if she were actually saying, I feel great. I can go out and do anything. I am afraid of nothing. I feel good and secure. At the same time, Lisa had become far more feminine than she had been before as this fragile, insecure creature. To me, femininity has always indicated strength, character, and confidence; and I saw it now in Lisa.

Lisa's example points up something I feel is universally true: When you feel secure enough with yourself, with your body, then you are really free to be feminine and beautiful, to be yourself.

The wonderful thing about your body is that at no stage or age is it beyond being changed, and changed drastically. You can lose 50 pounds, even 100 or more. You can firm up your body and change your entire look. In a short period of time, you can assume an active role in the life that has been passing you by. You can become more attractive, vigorous, and self-confident—all by deciding to change the shape of your body and then following through with it.

Begin by fixing one idea firmly in your mind. Say it to yourself now and never forget it, *I can do anything I want with my body!* If you need more mass on your thighs because they are too thin, you can increase them. If you want to decrease your hips, your buttocks, or your waist, you can do that with proper diet and some elementary exercises. You can actually reshape your whole body into what you want it to be. There are only two requirements:

- That you know what you want;
- That you are willing to expend the effort to achieve it.

Mind and Body

You have to learn to think of your body and mind as a single unit. Too often, people do not; they look at their body as though it were a piece of luggage, a burden they must carry with them through life—for better or worse. They take their bodies for granted, never actually being aware of its individual parts unless they are under some kind of stress, such as fatigue or the pain of illness or injury. Then they regard that particular part of their body as a traitor, an enemy, something that causes them anguish and which they must somehow fight and conquer. They express their frustration and anger in statements like, "My body doesn't respond to exercise." "My legs give me trouble." "My neck is stiff." "My back aches."

If you get sore or stiff, or if you feel weak, perhaps your body is trying to tell you there's something wrong. It's saying, Something needs to be done. Feeling good is the same. Your body is telling you, Hey, thanks, that's what I needed. I feel great! It's a connection your mind has to make.

Athletes who perform best realize their feats don't just happen because of their body, strength, coordination, or skill. The first and most important part is played by their mind, which is often referred to as the psychic power of sports. The reason is this: The mind has to visualize completely and concretely whatever the body must do before the body can follow through effectively.

The only time your body can react and do anything, even to lift an arm, is when your brain tells it to do so. Therefore, if you are serious about changing your body, you have to start by changing your mind.

The body rarely does anything by accident. This is obviously true

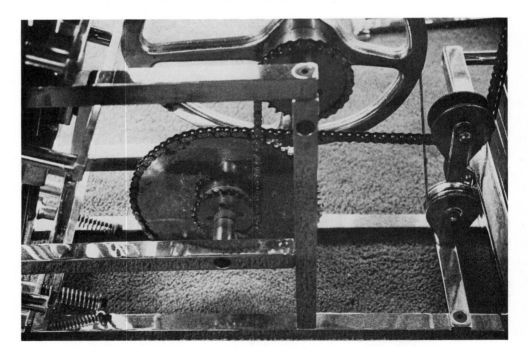

when it comes to breaking a world record or accomplishing some other seemingly superhuman task. If a weightlifter standing in front of a weight visualizes herself lifting the weight, then she can follow through and do it. The same with running. The runner has to decide she wants to break the world's record, and she has to believe in her decision. If she believes

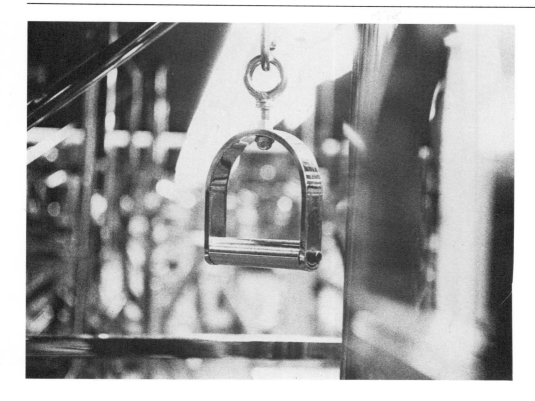

in it strongly enough, then she can do it. The mind gets the body going. In any type of physical endeavor, the mind is as important as the body.

Visualize yourself with the body you want. When you have fixed in your mind the image of the changed you, let that be your incentive for training and working out. This mental image should be your motivator, your goal, the ideal you are *determined* to reach. Now you can work systematically. For example, you can tell yourself, I must spend more time on my thighs, because in your vision your thighs are much smaller and smoother than now.

Your body and mind are one: two parts of a whole. They are you. Mind and body cannot and should not be separated. "If you are your body and your body is you," Alexander Lowen tells us in *Bioenergetics,* "then it expresses who you are. It is your way of being in the world. The more alive your body is, the more you are in the world. When your body loses some of its aliveness, as when you are exhausted, for example, you tend to withdraw."

Define how you want to improve your body. It isn't enough to say, I want to look better. Put it in words that can be measured and met in terms of solid goals. Tell yourself: I'm a size 12; I *want* to be a 10. My waist is 29 inches. I *want* to have a 26-inch waist. These are concrete terms your mind can comprehend.

After you have isolated the specific things you want to change, you must create willpower to carry through your desire, to get you to do the

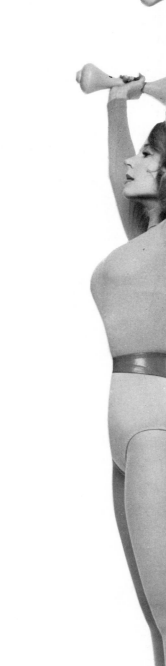

Betty Weider is living proof of how weight training keeps you young. Betty, who is in her mid-forties but looks mid-twenties, is married to Joe Weider, trainer of champions and publisher.

exercises in the first place and then keep you on your schedule. When you are confronted with ice cream or chocolate cake, it takes willpower to continue to see yourself as slim and to keep you from touching any of these garbage foods. Gradually, as you begin to see and feel results from exercise, maintaining your willpower will become easier.

As a regulator of the body, the mind is incredible. I learned, during years of training for bodybuilding contests, that once I had firmly established in my mind that I wanted certain goals, it was only a matter of time before I reached them.

This becomes a cycle I call the "confidence cycle." Once you see your body changing, you feel a sense of achievement and confidence. That, in turn, starts the mind believing it can do more and more. From there, the possibilities are almost limitless. Your mind must accept totally the image you've decided upon for a new body before you can make that body a reality and maintain it comfortably.

Work slowly. Set small goals at first; meet them; then set more difficult goals. Always—and this is essential—*always* acknowledge your progress regardless of how small it is. For instance, if you have set a goal to lose an inch from your waist or thighs in two weeks and you lose only three-quarters of an inch, do not say, I've failed. Look at it positively. Tell yourself, All right, I've already lost three-quarters of an inch. It was easy. This time I can lose an inch. Do not condition yourself to accept setbacks of any kind and never even remotely consider failure.

Now go ahead and become the person you want to be.

Age Doesn't Matter

When they pass the age of forty a lot of women make the mistake of thinking they will naturally look less attractive than they did when they were twenty. They say it is an inevitable part of aging. But what is really happening is that they are giving in, surrendering to aging.

Okay, they are saying. I'm getting older. I won't be as beautiful or as graceful as I once was. I don't care.

I believe they really do care. If a woman is strong and has pride in herself, if she likes herself and still has that vital spark, she will say, Wait a minute. I'm going to fight age. I won't accept it. Age can't take anything away from me. I am going to keep everything I have—my beauty, my flexibility, my active life, my energy, my strength and endurance.

There is no age at which you should not exercise, no point in life when it is too late to begin a systematic exercise program to rejuvenate yourself. In fact, the importance of exercise to your total well-being actually increases with age. Not that you will need *more* exercise, but as you grow older and less active, you therefore have a greater need for *planned* exercise—exercise designed to keep you stimulated and flexible —if you want to maintain full use of your bodily systems.

In his book, *Stress Without Distress,* Dr. Hans Selye maintains:

We have seen that unused muscles, brains, and other organs lose efficiency. To keep fit, we must exercise both our bodies and our minds. Besides, inactivity deprives us of every outlet for our innate urge to create, to build; this causes tensions and the insecurity that stems from aimlessness.

There is no way you can *save* your body by not using it. The result is just the opposite: Without use, your body atrophies. Exercise, especially exercise in a controlled program created to strengthen and maintain your entire body, can prevent and even overcome some of the ill effects of aging—neglected muscles, stiff joints and tendons, stooped shoulders, widow's hump, loose sagging upper arms, and the condition called *cellulite.* You can avoid these problems if you begin early in life to exercise regularly. But if you've already fallen victim to one or more of the above-mentioned results of bodily neglect—and chances are you have if you've allowed yourself to go for a number of years without proper exercise—you can begin to work now and gradually eliminate them.

Here are three basic rules I suggest you use in gauging my program to your age and current body condition:

1. If you are over thirty, have a complete physical checkup. Do not begin the exercises without it. Tell your doctor of your plans to begin working out, and then never do more than your doctor says you should do. (I will discuss this in greater detail later.)
2. Start slowly and increase your program gradually, taking care to master and become comfortable with all the movements of one exercise before you go on to a more advanced one.
3. Pay attention to what your muscles tell you. Never try to handle more weight or repetitions in any exercise than you can do without straining. Work hard, challenge yourself, but never overdo it.

Exercise will help your body in every way. It will make you feel more vital. Vitality is the key to a good life. With each exercise session, you will feel your vitality increase, and with it will come improvements in both your mental alertness and your sense of well-being.

A WORD OF CAUTION. If you've neglected your body for a long period, you will have to invest both time and effort to bring it back into shape. Be realistic about it. A twenty-year-old woman with very few physical problems is going to put in forty-five minutes to an hour three times a week, and in a month she will probably be in fantastic shape. On the other hand, a forty-year-old woman who has let herself go for twenty years may need to spend three or four months getting into the same shape. But it can and will happen. And three or four months of care (which is a total of no more than forty-eight actual hours of working out) is almost nothing compared to the twenty years of abuse and neglect your body might have suffered. But this is the marvelous thing about your body. No matter what condition it's in, it can be changed.

I can say from my own experience that the more I have exercised, the less I got ill. I was always sick as a child. But after I started participating in various sports and training with weights, I never again became seriously ill. A lot of women have remarked on the same thing. When they started

Better Health

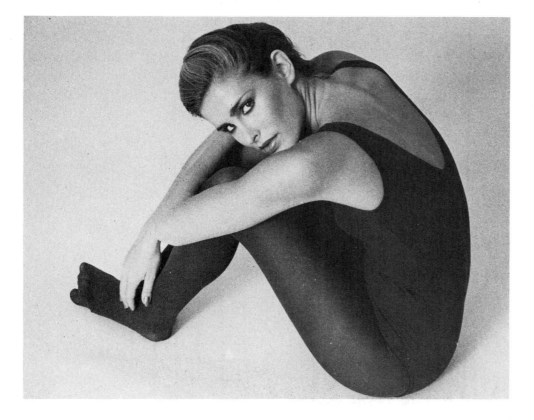

working out, they were only doing it for cosmetic reasons—losing a few inches around the thighs, firming up their breasts, or improving their calves. Better health is an unexpected fringe benefit of exercise. Along with feeling better and more active, many women in my fitness seminars state they have less troublesome menstrual periods; others say pregnancy and childbirth were both less complicated and less painful as a result of being in good physical condition.

Your own workouts should improve your general health, giving you positive results in all areas of your body—in your skeletal, pulmonary, cardiovascular, digestive, and nervous systems.

Due to stronger muscles and greater flexibility, your posture and carriage will become better. Your lungs will be strengthened, their capacity increased, making available more oxygen for your cells. Your heart will be stronger, your heart rate, and perhaps even your blood pressure, will be lowered, while its capacity and levels of efficiency will be raised. Improved circulation will provide more oxygen-rich blood for your tissues, increasing your overall energy level and passing on benefits to your skin, nails, and hair. The peristaltic action of your digestive system will be aided, helping to regulate your appetite and elimination and thereby giving you greater protection against disease in those and all other parts of your body.

Even your brain will benefit. Added oxygen to your brain cells increases their speed and efficiency, allowing you to be more alert and to have better reasoning powers. Regular exercise tends to relieve harmful stresses and anxieties responsible for fatigue and premature aging and will let you perform more efficiently on all levels.

Getting to Know Your Body

For the sake of convenience, we often divide human beings into three general body types: *ectomorph, mesomorph,* and *endomorph.* Some people have gone so far as calling these three types three different races —so different are they in appearance and in their way of approaching things.

Ectomorphs are often identified as thinkers. If you are an ectomorph, you are comparatively tall, willowy, with reedy bones, slender hands and fingers, narrow long feet, and a triangular-shaped face. Chances are, you've never had a weight problem. In fact, you may have a problem keeping on as much weight as you like or need. Because you tend to keep to yourself, you are likely to begin training alone or with a good friend.

Mesomorphs—the doers—are more athletic. If you fit this body type, you will be naturally muscular, sinewy, with broad, strong bones. You are probably inclined toward sports—tennis, swimming. There will be a certain boyishness to your figure and a square, determined look to your face. You will normally be ahead of the others in the gym.

Endomorphs are the talkers. Voluptuous will usually describe you when you are at your best weight and condition (which is probably not often enough). You are full of curves and round lines. Weight will be a concern to you. You've probably been on almost every diet devised by mankind. But you probably like to eat too much for your own good. Watch yourself. Exercise will not come naturally to you. When you start to tire, you may find yourself talking too much, joking, killing time you should be using to exercise.

One of the different body types isn't necessarily better than another. One may have a few more advantages in sports or training, but all three have their own problems, and in each case the problem can be corrected. It is the same in professional bodybuilding. I've had skinny men come into the gymnasium thinking: I'll never have the chance of being a big muscular guy because I'm not the right body type. I tell them their size doesn't matter; they just have to approach things differently.

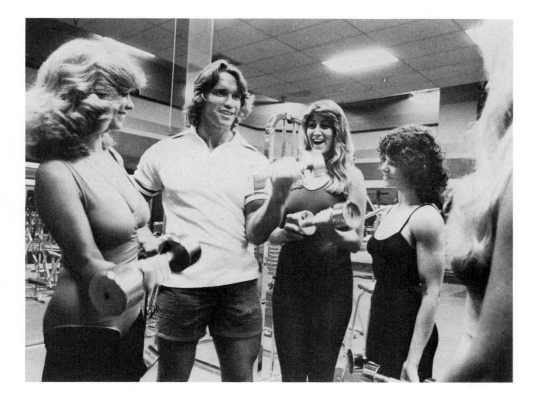

They need to make their bodies grow with a quick-gain diet and do more exercises to build up certain weak areas. They have to adjust their training and eating habits, and they can end up in the same class with the bigger guys. Maybe it won't be as easy, but it can still be done. In bodybuilding, men like Frank Zane and Franco Columbu had all the disadvantages when they started. They were slim and bony, but they ended up being Mr. Universe. Exactly the opposite was true of Bruce Randall, who weighed 400 pounds, cut down to 198 pounds, and won Mr. Universe, too.

Women can change as dramatically. Those who are too skinny—the ectomorphs—can build lean muscle tissue and improve the shape of their bodies. The endomorphs can go on a diet and a vigorous training routine, and trim their bodies to become smoother, lighter, sexier. Instead of stuffing themselves with food, they'll have to learn to eat less, and those who are skinny and never eat much may have to start eating more. But every woman has the potential of reshaping her body and

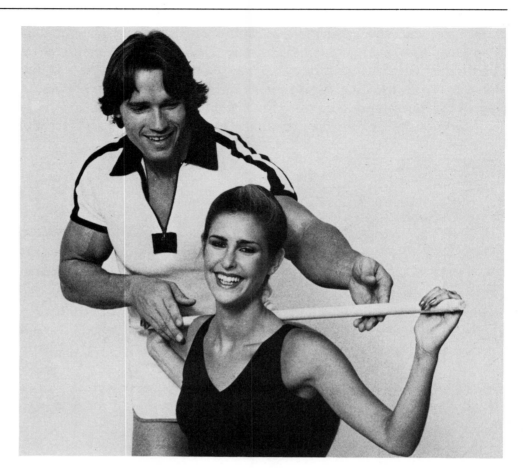

becoming beautiful as long as she has a strong vision in her mind of what she wants to look like. That, finally, is the only thing that really counts.

It's often easier just to accept your weaknesses and your faults, physically and mentally, to make excuses and learn to live with yourself —with your fat, your saggy breasts, your cellulite. But it's totally contrary to what I believe. You should not accept shortcomings to be with you forever. You should fight them and you can overcome them. You should take control.

If you watch a woman who is in control, no matter where she is— at home, in the street, at a party—she handles herself with beauty and grace. She radiates confidence and moves easily, seeming to flow from room to room, from place to place. And the attention she gets builds her ego, which boosts her self-confidence. With self-confidence, she becomes more convincing, and her outlook on life becomes more positive. The result is that her life just gets better and better.

The worst thing you can do to undermine yourself is to justify being out of shape. "I don't like parties," "I don't like to dance," or "I hate going to the beach." What this really tells us is that the person making these excuses is not being honest with herself. If you are full of such empty excuses, sit down and analyze why you make them. Why don't I want to go to a party? Why don't I want to go dancing? Why don't I want to go to the beach? Does it have anything to do with the places or the functions themselves, or is it really that you don't want to be in public because of the way you look?

Do not be depressed and, above all, do not accept it as your fate. Do something about it. Change yourself.

Self-Appraisal

Purchase a notebook in which you can record all your personal data (height, measurements, weight), your observations, your progress, and periodic evaluations of yourself. As this is to be a permanent record, choose a sturdy notebook from which pages cannot be torn out or replaced. The idea is to accept yourself as you are now, complete with faults and shortcomings. Only then can you be objective about the changes you want to make. Now, stand before the mirror and undress. This may be difficult. Many people get out of bed and immediately put on their bathrobe. As soon as they're out of the shower, they dry themselves and wrap themselves in a big towel. They are constantly hiding. I know it will be difficult for some of you to undress, look at yourself, and acknowledge something you haven't wanted to face for years: cellulite, varicose veins, dead-looking skin, saggy breasts, or mottled buttocks. Just remember, there is no reason to become depressed; you know you can change your body and this should motivate you.

Edith Head, the Hollywood designer, suggests you take a large brown paper bag, cut out two eyeholes, and then place it over your

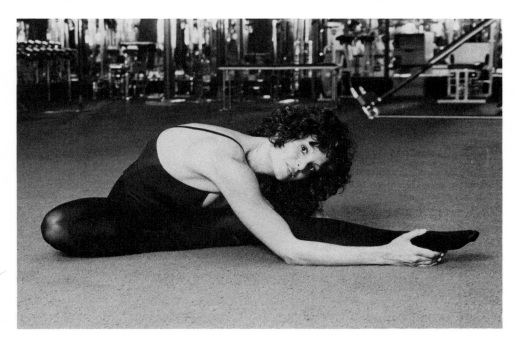

head. Her reasoning is that if you can't see your face in the mirror, you can be much more objective. Try it and see if it doesn't work for you.

Take off your clothing slowly, one garment at a time. Watch yourself in the mirror. How do you look when you bend? Are your movements as liquid as you would like them to be? Do you see areas of your body where you seem to have fallen apart? Are the lines still as good as they once were?

When you are fully undressed, take a few moments and look at yourself from the front. Be thorough, make a mental note of everything you see.

Turn to the side. Check the side view carefully. Turn the other way. Is there a difference?

Face away from the mirror and, looking back over your shoulder with a small hand mirror, examine how you look from behind. Don't allow your eyes to flit over any area that is displeasing. Study it. Evaluate it. How would you improve it?

With your notebook, sit in full view of the mirror. Look at yourself

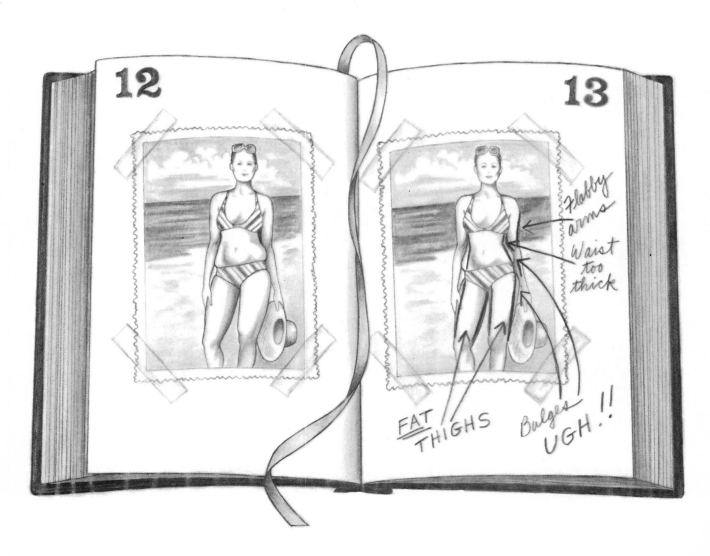

frequently and write your impressions. Be as detached, objective, and honest as you can. Your honesty in the beginning will help you set your goals and motivate you to correct your problems in the weeks and months to come.

It may be necessary to get up a few times and look at yourself in the mirror—just to make sure you are being neither too harsh nor too lenient. Note the lines of your waist, buttocks, thighs, and the flesh just above your knees—front and back. Are the curves smooth and pleasing to the eye?

Do not be afraid to write about your good as well as your bad points. If you like the looks of your legs or your breasts, say so; tell yourself why. Be explicit. I believe all criticism should be constructive; it should be geared to producing positive results.

Standing before the mirror again, examine yourself thoroughly, limb by limb. Touch yourself. Grab the extra flesh. Feel the folds of fat. Note where your skin is slack—take hold and give it a good tug. Go over every inch of your body as if you were examining another person, as if

26

Weight: last week – 135
this week – 130
Goals for next week:
1) More repetitions in everything except push-ups
2) Trim one more inch from waist
3) Eat only fresh fruit for dessert

BIG GOAL

Be size 10 again in one month!

27

General observations:
Worst areas are still thighs and stomach. Work! Work!

Arms are firming up nicely –

Finally got into last years jeans !!

another person were examining you. Write down both your findings and your reactions. Then tell yourself how beautiful you are going to look, as you exercise and realize the ideal image you have set for yourself.

Your Scales, Tape Measure, and Mirror

Weight should not be the criterion by which you evaluate your progress. In the beginning, you can lose 3 or 4 inches from your waist by exercising and dieting and still not see that much loss on the scale. Why? Because in doing the exercises, you will have built up a number of muscles, and the density and weight of this new muscle tissue is much greater than an equivalent mass of fat. You should weigh yourself, of course, and keep a record of it. But I urge you to concentrate more on the visual picture of yourself than on what your scales tell you.

Make a chart, such as the one below, in your notebook. Measure yourself and write the results in the appropriate blanks. At the end of each week, make a new chart and keep an accurate record of your progress.

	MEASUREMENTS	GOAL
upper arm	_____	_____
chest	_____	_____
bustline	_____	_____
waistline	_____	_____
hips	_____	_____
buttocks	_____	_____
right thigh	_____	_____
left thigh	_____	_____
right calf	_____	_____
left calf	_____	_____

Take three photographs of yourself—front, back, side—in order to have a photographic record of your present state of fitness. Make two copies of each. A nude photograph is best, but if you absolutely cannot bring yourself to it, then you can get by with one in a tight-fitting bathing suit or a snug, flesh-colored leotard. The whole procedure can be handled with ease if you own or borrow an automatic camera that will develop the film instantly. Set the camera on a tripod or some other sturdy support, use the self-timer, and photograph yourself.

Glue both sets of photographs on opposite pages of your notebook —either before or immediately after the observations you have just made about yourself. Leave the first set untouched. Then, with a fine-pointed grease pencil or china marker, mark on each photograph of the second set exactly how you *want* to look. Trim off any bulges, nip in here and there, curve and mold: Use the grease pencil the way you will be using the exercises.

Write something in your notebook each workout day. Record your progress; set down new goals. Write how you feel about what the exercise is doing to your body and how it is changing your overall feeling about yourself. At the beginning of each exercise program and at regular intervals—two weeks, a month—take new photographs. Compare them to the first photographs you took, the ones you left untouched, as well as the ones you marked. This should help you see the changes you have made and push you ahead to accomplishing new goals.

For your own peace of mind, keep this notebook private. When you finish writing each daily exercise in it, keep it in a safe, private place such as your lingerie drawer. The danger of sharing it with people is you may find them either laughing about it or making negative comments, which could be discouraging.

Whatever else you may do, keep a notebook. It has been proven that you're more likely to accomplish goals if you've written them down. Your notebook can serve as an accurate gauge of your progress. From its pages, you'll be able to see how much you have changed with each month of training.

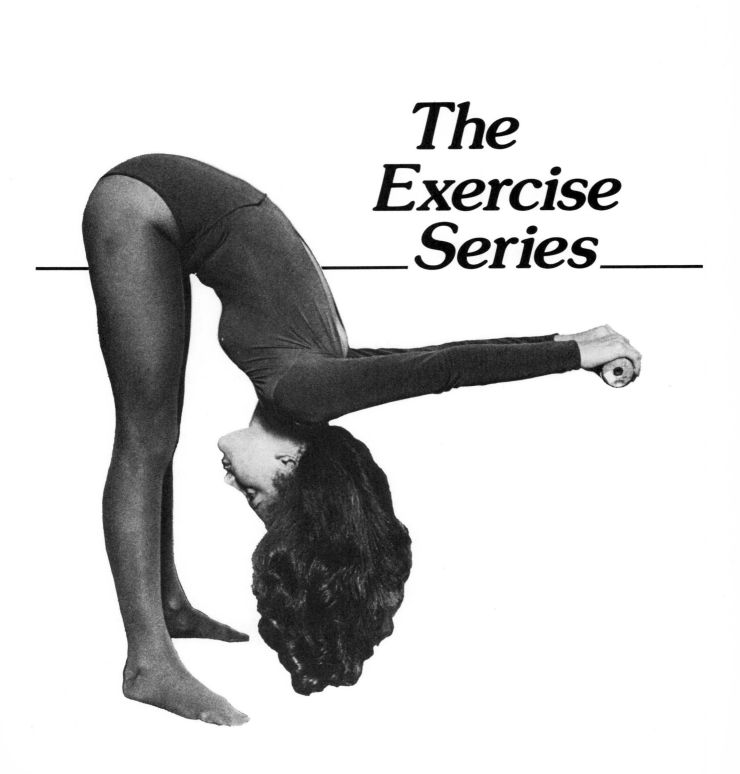

The
Exercise
Series

SERIES 1

Introductory Resistance Exercises

These at-home exercises utilize the natural resistance of your own body weight to help you shape up, increase muscle tone, and achieve more flexibility. Two exercises with lightweight dumbbells are included to prepare you for the gym.

SERIES 2

Gymwork

This series provides a solid introduction to the gym and the gym equipment—the resistance machines—designed to isolate and thoroughly exercise each muscle group. The exercises are designed so you get the greatest return, the most benefit, out of each movement.

SERIES 3

Supersets

Supersetting is combining two exercises for related or complementary body parts and doing them back to back with no rest interval between them. It is an advanced, sophisticated, and very strenuous program for the really enthusiastic.

SERIES 4

Exercises for Anytime, Anyplace

This program is for the woman who travels or cannot get to a gym and is included so that you have no excuse not to work out. It is an advanced program beyond the introductory resistance exercises.

EACH SERIES is made up of exercises that should be done in the order indicated. Start each exercise session with the warm-up routine described on page 48 and finish with the stretches that are described directly after.

To make the workouts as beneficial as they can be, you have to learn to breathe properly during exercise. Basically, the rule is to exhale when you encounter most resistance and inhale when you encounter the least resistance. A good example is a push-up from the floor: As you push up—the moment of most resistance—you exhale; then, as you let yourself back down to the floor—the movement of least resistance— you inhale. At first, controlling your breathing will take a conscious effort, but gradually it will become natural to you. Breathing instructions accompany each exercise.

The number of repetitions are also indicated for each exercise. A repetition is one complete movement of an exercise—one whole push-up, one bench press, one curl, etc. Don't force yourself if you can't do all of them; work gradually to achieve the number I have specified. The reps or repetitions should follow one another smoothly and rhythmically, without breaks between. It may take time to familiarize yourself sufficiently with the exercises and become flexible enough to be able to maintain this rhythm. You will find that exercises done in a rhythmical pattern will leave you feeling exhilarated and energized. Exercises done jerkily to an indefinite pattern will drain your energy store and leave you feeling exhausted.

A set, as opposed to a rep, is the number of repetitions done in succession. If an exercise works first one arm or leg and then the other arm or leg, and the directions call for ten repetitions, you should do ten repetitions for *each* arm or leg to complete a single set. If two sets are specified, do the number of repetitions called for, rest briefly, then repeat. Unless otherwise indicated, a set should take no longer than 1 minute. One reason to work out in sets is because muscles respond best to a pattern of being worked, rested, then worked again. The exceptions are the abdominal, waist, and calf muscles.

The ideal number of sets is given for each exercise as is the number of pounds—the amount of weight—in those exercises where weights are indicated.

BEFORE YOU BEGIN. Everyone needs exercise. Every body regardless of its age or condition will benefit from resistance training. However, there are people with certain physical conditions that make it inadvisable to do certain kinds of exercise. Before you embark upon any exercise program, go to your physician for a complete checkup. Prior to the examination, tell your doctor what you plan to do and ask for a go-ahead. If you have a problem, the doctor can work with you to correct it, tell you how to pace yourself, and advise you on avoiding certain exercises. Most of you will get an absolute go-ahead. But there may be a few who will be cautioned to go more slowly and work up to the full program.

SET A REGULAR TIME FOR EXERCISE. Spend only 45 minutes to an hour a day three times a week working out. These blocks of time are significant and meaningful and should be kept regular and consistent. Do not change them. You will achieve the best results if you space your exercise sessions so there is a full day between them, for example, Monday, Wednesday, Friday.

Exercise for at least 45 minutes but never longer than an hour, *never* more than three times a week. In fact, once your session is over, don't even think about exercise until the next one is due. Continue to run, swim, play tennis, but don't devise ways to turn the other hours of your life into exercise times. I'm talking about things like running up two stairs at a time, doing a stiff-legged toe-touch each time you bend over to pick up something you dropped. Do the exercises I have outlined with a definite goal in mind, then enjoy the rest of your life.

EXERCISE IS NOT PUNISHMENT. When you first start training, you should not treat your body as though it deserves punishment for being in poor condition. You will make yourself sore and become turned off to the whole idea of working out. Remember, you are introducing your body to something new. So you should take it easy; go at it step by step. Listen to your body and stay in touch with it.

I recommend that you train with each exercise series at least one month. Make sure you are comfortable with all the exercises and variations of one series before you move on to the next. If it takes two months, or even three, that's fine. DO NOT SPEND LESS THAN A MONTH. If the exercises become too easy, increase the weight or add another set.

IN YOUR NOTEBOOK, write down all the data pertinent to the exercises themselves—how many repetitions you do, how many sets, how much weight you use. In addition, describe your feelings about the exercises, what is happening to your body, and how your attitude about it is changing. State your goals and the date you accomplish them. If you fall short of a goal, try to figure out why. At the beginning and end of each series, take a new photograph of yourself. Compare it to the previous ones.

EXERCISE TO MUSIC. In the last few years, I've noticed more and more women's gymnasiums are using music as an aid to exercise. I believe this practice has a lot of advantages. Music itself is a terrific motivator for body movement. The beat of the music establishes a rhythm, which is good for working out, good for the body. The body itself is governed by rhythmical patterns—the regular beat of the heart, the flow of the blood, breathing. Music, because it reduces monotony, can also help you relax and get more out of each exercise. So whether you train at home or in a gymnasium, try to do it to music. The records or tapes ought to be chosen not for their serene qualities, but for a strong definite beat that will keep you moving at a smooth, fairly fast pace.

Music and Exercise

WHAT TO WEAR. Choose clothes for your workouts in which you feel good. They should be comfortable and allow you to move without restriction. Natural fibers, especially cotton, will feel better against your skin than synthetic ones. Cotton absorbs perspiration, dries quickly, and is easy to care for.

Warm-Ups

Begin each exercise session with a few minutes of warm-up to increase your heart rate and pump blood out to your muscles, where it will be needed. Use this warm-up time to whet your enthusiasm and prepare your mind for your workout.

Start the music and begin moving in half-time. Stretch all your limbs. Do 4 or 5 knee bends. Reach for the sky 3 times with each arm. Touch your toes slowly 5 times. Rotate your neck twice in each direction. Bend backward 4 times. Run in place for 10 seconds. Do 5 kicks, alternately, with each leg.

Now pick up a lightweight dumbbell with both hands and stand with your feet approximately 12 inches apart. Hold the dumbbell out in front of you, at shoulder height. Keeping both arms straight, lift the dumbbell slowly above your head; then bring it smoothly down between your legs and as far back as you can. All through the movement, keep your elbows and knees locked.

Holding the dumbbell out at waist level and keeping your hips and legs stationary, swing your arms as far as you can to the right, then back around and as far as you can to the left.

Hold the dumbbell shoulder height, as in the first movement. Stand with your feet approximately 12 inches apart. Raise up on tiptoe. Remaining on your toes, squat down until your thighs are parallel to the floor, as in the photograph. Lift yourself slowly to a full standing position.

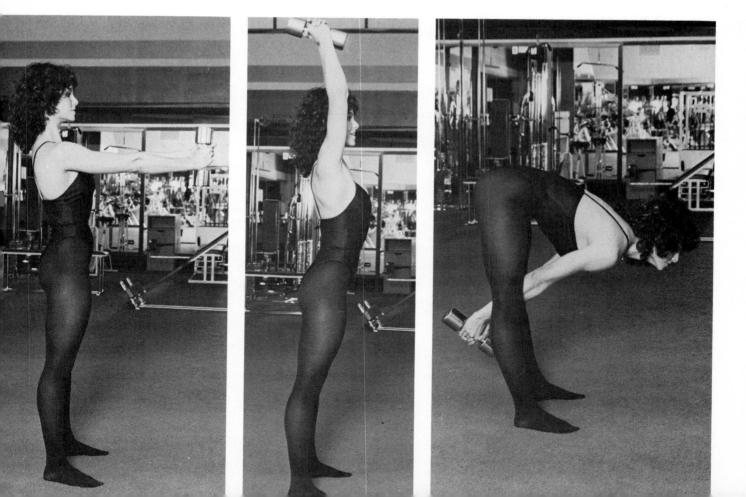

End each exercise session with some stretching movements. Stretching is essential for proper development and toning. By elongating the muscle tissues, you allow the blood to flow freely through them, which keeps them loose and limber and which, in turn, makes you feel relaxed, refreshed, and helps relieve tension.

Begin from a sitting position—your legs in a wide-stride split, your right knee bent, your left leg straight.

Grasp the ankle of your left leg with both hands and pull your head down to touch your left knee. Stretch the pelvis in this movement by bringing it as near as you can to your thigh. Return to a sitting position.

Extend your left hand over your head and brace your right hand on the floor next to your right knee. Now lift your body up onto your right knee and stretch your left arm over your head. Hold the extreme position for a few seconds to feel the resistance.

When done properly, this is a total body stretch. Repeat 10 times on each side.

Stretches

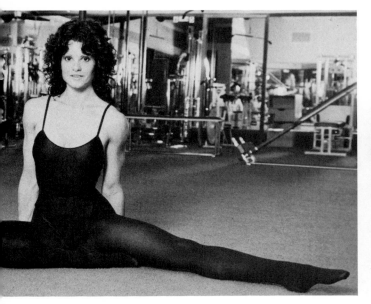

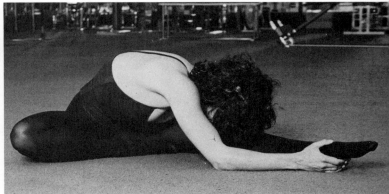

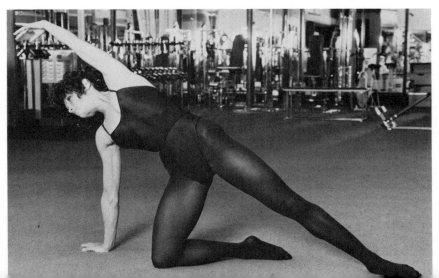

When the beginning stretching movements have become easy, add this Three-Way Stretch to your program.

The basic position: Sit on the floor with legs spread as far as possible. (Within a few days, you should be able to increase it by a few inches.) Stretch both hands as far down your legs as you can, trying to reach the ankles. Hold for a count of 10. Relax. This will be the basic leg position for all three movements of the exercise.

The first movement: Lean forward, grasp your left ankle lightly, and pull your torso gently toward your left foot. Don't strain, but be sure you feel the stretch in the muscles all along your right side. Straighten up and rest for a moment in the basic position. Do the same thing on the right side, resting in the center position each time. Alternating from side to side, start with 10 to each side, increasing to 20.

The second movement: Begin by extending your left hand across your abdomen and clasping your right thigh. Then curl your right arm

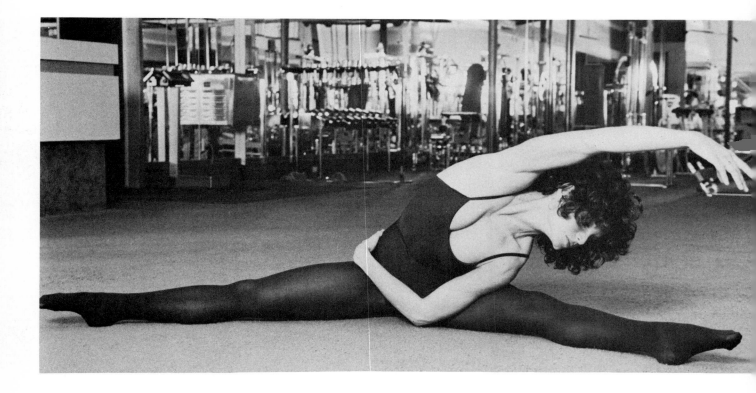

gracefully over your head, bending your torso to the left side, and try to touch your shoulder to your thigh. Hold for a count of 10. Alternating from side to side, start with 10 to each side, increasing to 20.

The third movement: This is possibly the most difficult progression of the Three-Way Stretch. Extend both arms gracefully in the air above your head. Now stretch as far as you can to the left, bringing your left elbow as close to your left leg as possible. Hold for a count of 10. Straighten up slowly. Now do the same thing to the right side. Alternating from side to side, start with 10 to each side, increasing to 20.

Stretch your muscles wherever you feel they need it. Spend some time experimenting with your body, working on the areas that are stiff.

Another good stretching movement that works similar to the Three-Way Stretch is the Elevated Leg Stretch. Place your left leg on a table. Bend forward and touch your hands and head to your leg, keeping both legs straight. Repeat with the right leg on the table.

Simple toe-touches—where you bend down and touch your toes, holding the position for a few counts while keeping the knees locked—alternated with reaching for the sky are also excellent stretch movements.

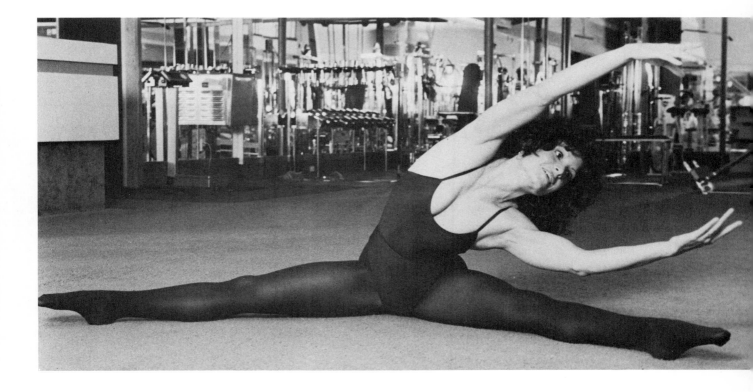

SERIES 1
Introductory Resistance Exercises

THESE FREEHAND EXERCISES are designed to be done at home. What you will need is a clear area of floor—an exercise mat or a padded carpet will make it more comfortable and prevent bruises—a chair, a broomstick or mopstick, and a set of lightweight dumbbells—3 to 5 lbs. I suggest you work out in front of a mirror if you can. This will help you stay in touch with yourself, achieve correct form, and let you see how much you are progressing.

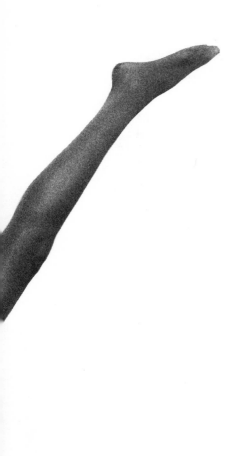

LEG LIFT

PURPOSE: To firm and trim the outer thigh.

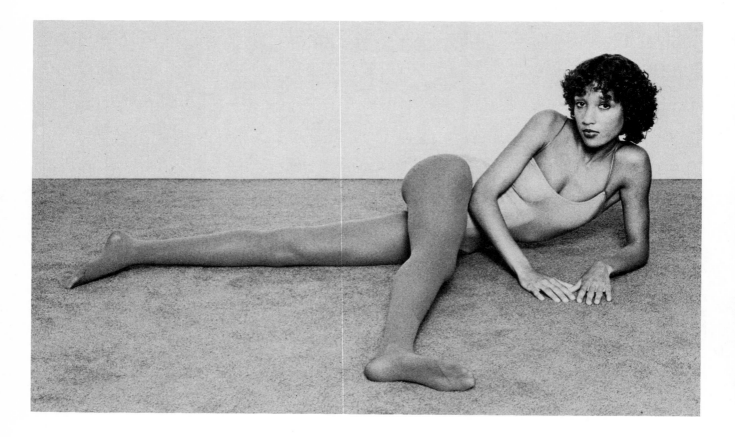

Lie on your left side with your left leg straight and the right (or top) leg at a right angle to the left (or bottom) leg, which should be kept in a straight line with your body. Support yourself by placing your elbow and hands firmly on the floor.

Raise your right leg up and lower down in a smooth movement, always maintaining the same right-angle position. Your hip should remain in a constantly flexed position as you use the muscles of the outer thigh to lift the leg. Note: Keep your foot parallel to the floor and

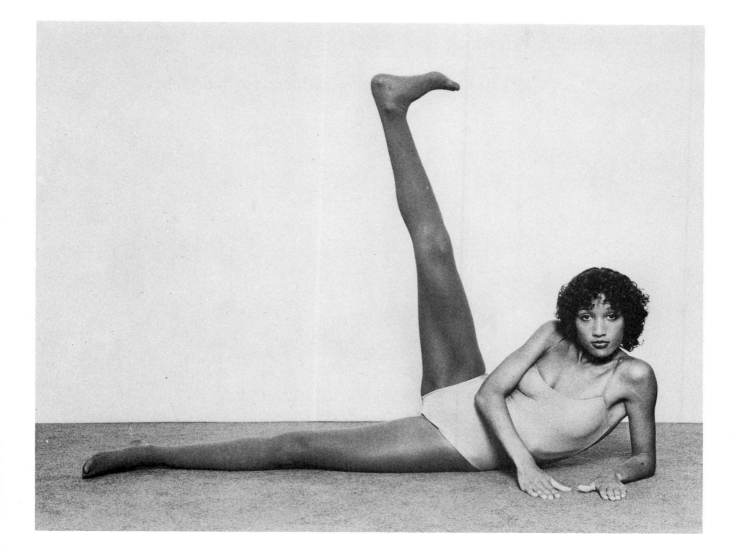

avoid pointing your toes because if your foot is rotated out of position, the wrong muscles will be worked. See photograph.

Turn and repeat the sequence with your other leg.

BREATHING: Inhale as you lift leg; exhale as you lower leg.
REPS: 10 to 15, working up to 50 in two weeks
SETS: 2, increasing to 3 in fourth week

SCISSOR LEG LIFT

PURPOSE: To trim and tighten the inner thigh.

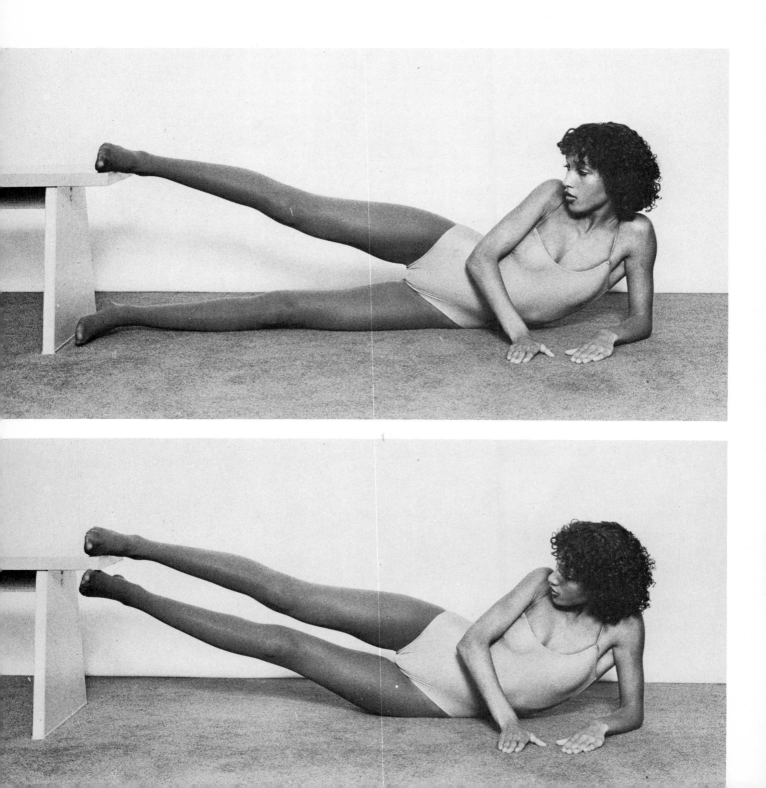

Lying on your left side, lift your right foot up; rest it on a bench or chair seat, keeping your leg straight.

Then bring your left foot up to meet your right foot, pause, and let it slowly and smoothly back to the floor. This creates the scissor effect which works the muscles of your inner thigh. Remember, only your left leg should move.

Turn and repeat the exercise with your right leg.

BREATHING: Exhale as you lift leg; inhale as you lower it.

REPS: 10 with each leg, increase to 50. Note: If you continue to have a problem with loose inner thighs, as many women have, increase the number of repetitions to 100.

SETS: 2, increasing to 3 in fourth week

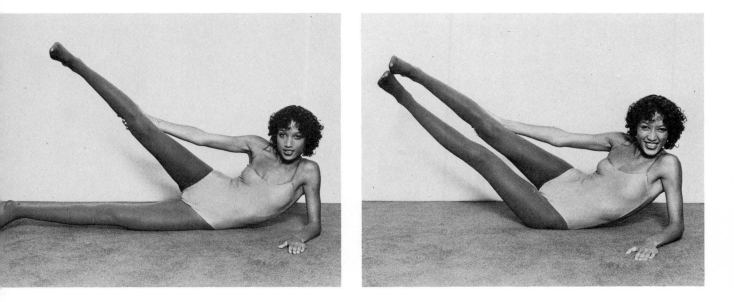

As you become more comfortable with the movements of this exercise, you can make it more difficult by holding the elevated leg with your arm instead of placing it on a bench.

REAR LEG LIFT

PURPOSE: To reduce and tighten the buttocks.

Kneel; with your elbows on the floor, hold your hands together and lace your fingers to form a "V" into which you place your head. Keeping your right knee on the floor, extend your left leg until it is straight out behind you. Pause, then bring your leg back to the beginning position.

Next, keeping your left knee on the floor, extend your right leg, and repeat the lifting movements. Alternate, lifting left leg, then right.

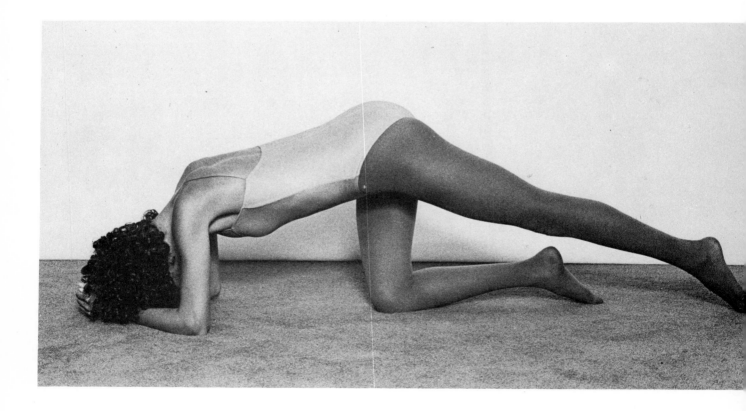

BREATHING: Exhale as you lift your leg; inhale as you lower your
leg.
REPS: 10 to 15 for each leg, working up to 30 or 40
SETS: 2, increasing to 3 in the fourth week

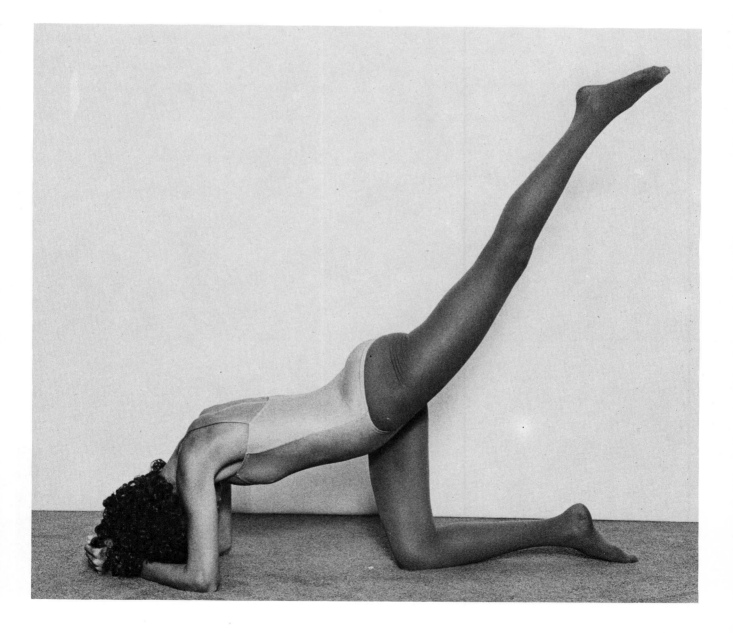

ELEVATED LEG CRUNCHES

PURPOSE: To firm up the abdomen and trim the waist.

Most exercises for the abdomen are also good for the legs because the quadriceps (the muscles in your frontal thighs) extend up and attach onto the pelvis. So this exercise will benefit two different areas of your body—the abdomen and the front of the thighs.

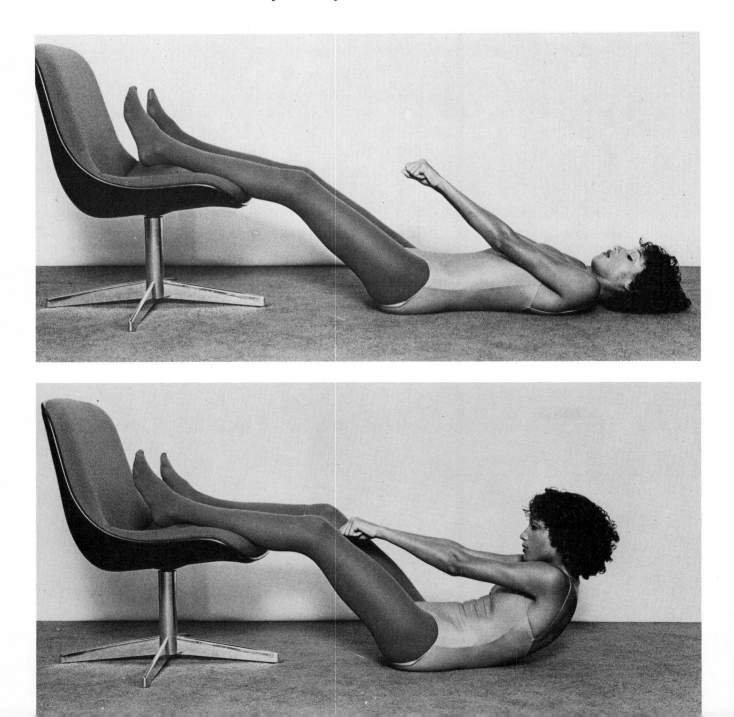

To start, lie flat on the floor with your calves resting on a chair or bench. Make fists and extend your arms above your body.

Moving slowly, bring your head, shoulders, and arms as far forward as possible. Your legs shouldn't move. And you shouldn't use your arms to give you momentum. Try lifting your shoulders forward without any help from your arms.

Elevated Leg Crunches do not require much movement. The idea is to crunch the muscles together, not to stretch them. By raising your legs, you work your lower abdominal muscles; and by lifting your shoulders forward, you work your upper abdominal muscles. You'll be able to feel this after a few repeititons.

Move slowly during this exercise and work up to as many repetitions as you can do in 2 or 3 minutes.

BREATHING: Exhale as you lift your body; inhale as you lie back.
REPS: 30–50
SETS: 2, increasing to 3 in the fourth week

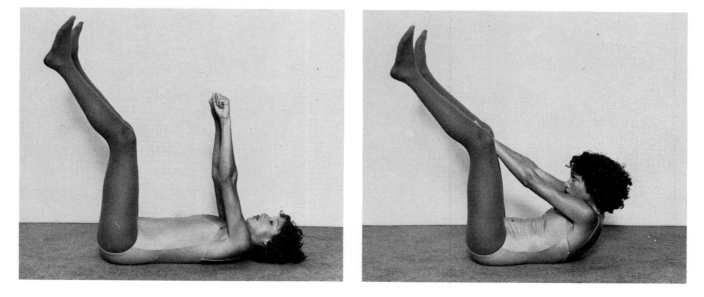

As you find this exercise easier to do, you can move on to the more difficult position. Instead of resting your legs on a chair, lift them in the air, keeping your knees slightly bent and spread approximately 12 to 14 inches. Try to imagine your toes are actually tied by a string to some point on the ceiling and you do not want to break the string. Moving slowly, lift your shoulders and push your hands as far as you can between your knees. Do as many as you can in 3 minutes.

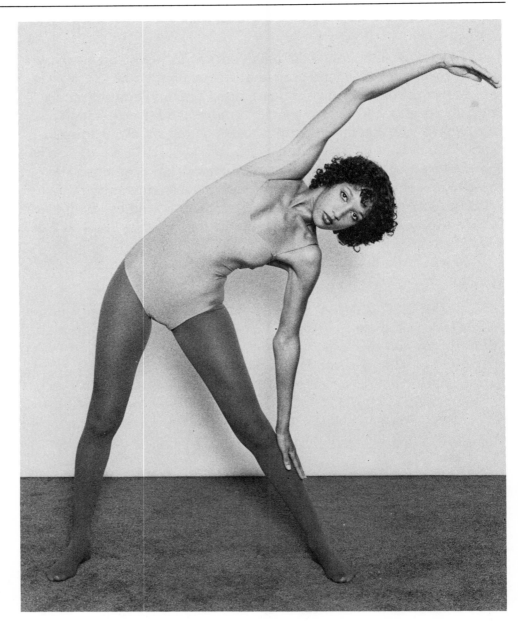

WAIST SLIMMER

PURPOSE: To slenderize muscles in the sides of the waist.

The Waist Slimmer, which is done in two movements, is designed to work the obliques—the muscles that crisscross the side of your waist. This exercise has a nice flowing rhythm, and once you've mastered its movements, you'll feel terrific doing it.

Stand with your feet 3 feet apart. Let your left hand rest on your thigh and raise your right arm in the air. Now bend to the left until your left hand slides down and touches your calf. Hold this extreme position to the count of 10.

Bend to the right, raising your left arm in the air and pushing your left hand down to touch your calf. Hold to the count of 10. Each time you go from one side to the other, grasp your calf lightly. Try not to bend forward while doing this movement; that way you'll work the obliques to their utmost. Hold the extreme position as long as possible.

BREATHING: Exhale as you bend to the side.
REPS: 25 to each side
SETS: 2, increasing to 3 in the fourth week

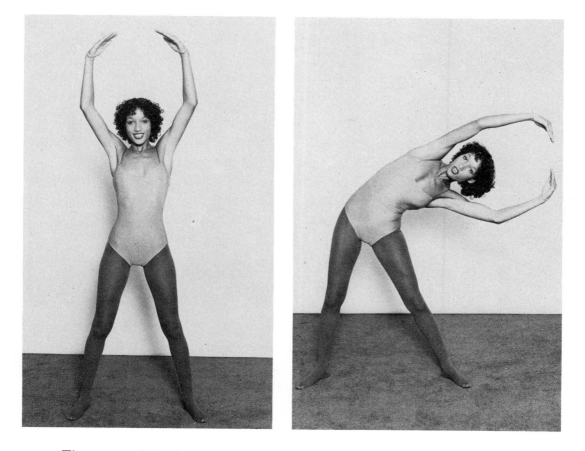

This more difficult movement should be started as soon as the other becomes easy. Raise both arms in the air in a very graceful, almost dancelike position. Move from side to side, going down as far as you can.

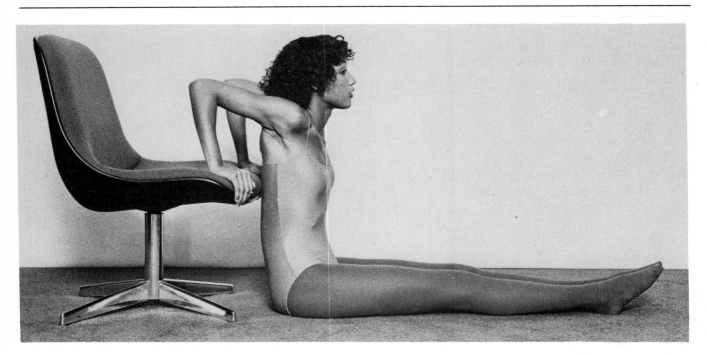

TRICEPS PUSH-UP

PURPOSE: To firm up the back part of your upper arm.

With women of any age, one of the weakest parts of their body is the triceps, the muscles in the back of the upper arm. Unless a woman is engaged in a great deal of pushing and pulling, she rarely uses her triceps. This accounts for those sagging muscles and fat deposits at the back of the arms. The triceps push-up will eliminate that problem by reducing fat and toning up the muscles.

The triceps push-up works directly on the triceps. It puts the shoulder in such a position that both ends of the triceps are exercised along with the anterior deltoids, which will help smooth your shoulders.

As a prop, you can use a chair, bench, stool, low table, or sturdy hassock. Choose one that seems the correct height for your particular body size (this will probably change as you increase in flexibility). Sit with your legs extended straight out in front of you and your back almost touching the prop. Lift your hands up behind you and grip the prop, keeping your fingers pointed toward your body.

Push your body up until your arms are straight and the elbows are locked. Again, ease your body slowly back to the floor; the negative resistance can be almost as effective as pushing up. As you become more adept at this exercise and your body becomes limber, you can increase the height of the prop and create more resistance.

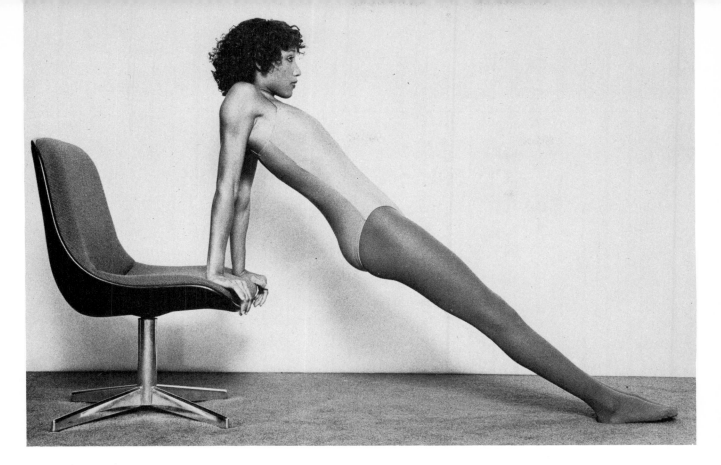

If you are unable to do the triceps push-up from the chair, do a triceps press from the floor, below.

BREATHING: Exhale as you push up; inhale as you let your body back to the floor.

REPS: 10, working up to 25

SETS: 2, increasing to 3 in the fourth week

Lie on the floor with your elbows bent behind you and your fingers pointing along the line of your body.

Lift your body up until your arms are straight. Hold. Then let your body slowly back to the floor. Move only your arms and torso during the movements of this exercise. As soon as this exercise becomes easy, go to the Triceps Push-up above.

BREATHING: Exhale as you push up from the floor; inhale as you lower yourself back.

REPS: 10, working up to 20

SETS: 2, increasing to 3 in the fourth week

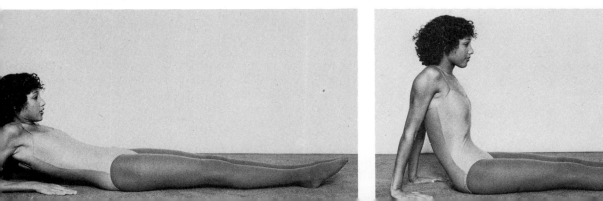

PUSH-UPS FROM THE KNEES

PURPOSE: To firm and increase the bustline.

The best way of keeping your breasts firm is to build up the pectoral muscles which span the breastplate and underlie the breast tissue and glands. The push-up is the most successful freehand exercise to really work these muscles.

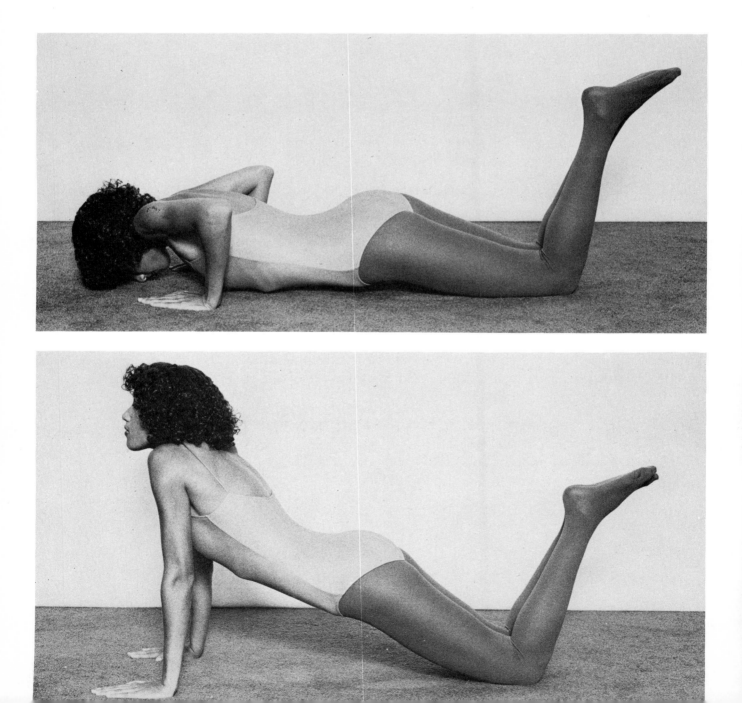

I want to emphasize that by building up the pectorals, you will probably improve the look of your breasts—even add an inch or two to the overall measurement of your bustline—but you are not likely to affect the size of the breasts themselves.

Lie flat on the floor face down, knees bent, and place your hands on the floor at shoulder width. Raise your body with your arms. When your arms are straight, pause; then lower your body to the floor, allowing only your chest to touch.

BREATHING: Exhale as you lift your body; inhale as you let it down.
REPS: 10
SETS: 2, increasing to 3 in the fourth week

If you are unable to do the push-ups from the knees, start with push-ups from the pelvis. Besides working the pectorals, push-ups from the pelvis also condition the back and the triceps. Note: If you must begin with push-ups from the pelvis, try, after a week, to move on to push-ups from the knees.

Lie face down on the floor, keeping your legs straight and together. Using the same hand position as you would for push-ups from the knees, push your torso up with your arms.

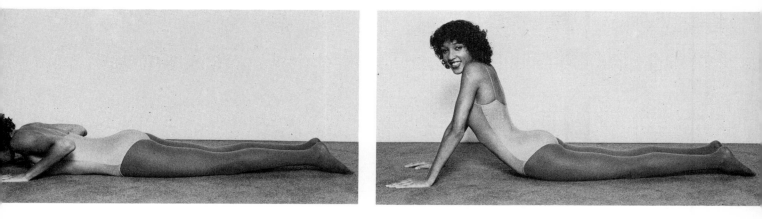

Note: No matter how you do push-ups—from the knees or from the pelvis—or how many you are able to do, the most important thing to remember is to do them correctly, which means lifting your body only with your arms. One good, well-executed push-up is more effective than 10 incorrect push-ups. When you can do one well, I know you will gradually be able to increase the number of repetitions.

CALF RAISES

PURPOSE: To firm, trim, or build the calves.

To have beautiful legs, a woman must have beautiful, well-shaped calves. And the best exercise to help build, decrease, or maintain your calves is Calf Raises.

Stand on a thick book or a block of wood, supporting and balancing your body by holding on to the back of a chair. Your toes should be on the book, your heels on the floor.

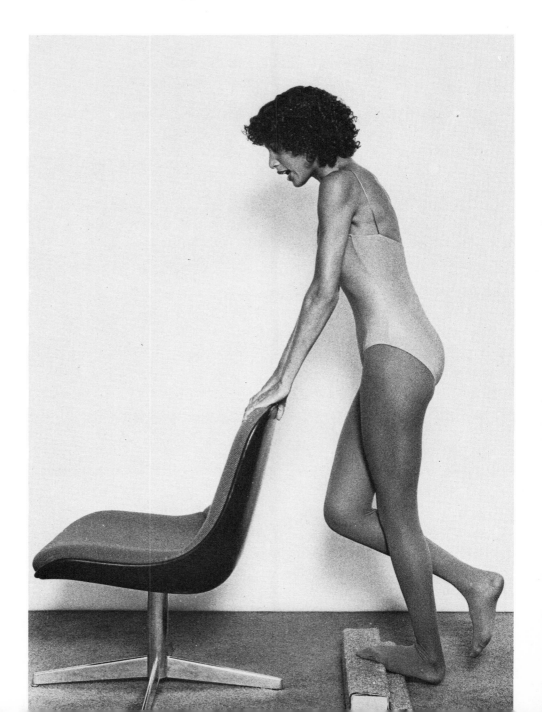

Starting with your left leg, raise the heel off the floor as far as possible until you're fully up on tiptoe. Slowly lower your heel back down to the floor. While you are lifting and lowering yourself with your left leg, your right leg should remain bent at the knee and relaxed.

BREATHING: Exhale as you go up on your toes; inhale as you come down.

REPS: 10 to 15 for each leg, working up to 30 within two weeks

SETS: 2

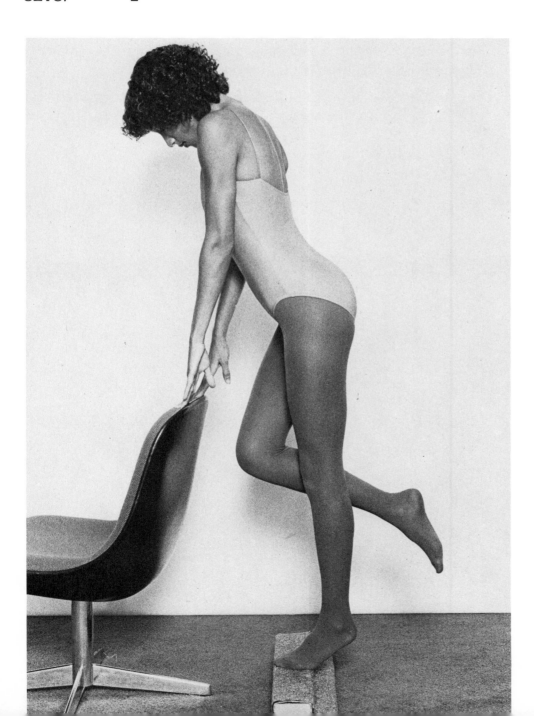

PULL-UPS BETWEEN CHAIRS

PURPOSE: To tone muscles in the back and shoulders.

Place two chairs back to back about 4 feet apart, and rest a broomstick across the backs of the two chairs. Lie flat on the floor, reach up, and grasp the broomstick, palms up, with your hands spread wide.

Holding your body perfectly straight, pull up, using only your arms. Keep your heels on the floor and don't allow them to move as you pull up.

As with push-ups from the knees, the important thing here is to do this exercise correctly, moving only your arms. Start with as many repetitions as possible, even if it is only one.

BREATHING: Exhale as you pull up; inhale as you lower yourself back to the floor.

REPS: 10

SETS: 3, increasing to 4 in the fourth week

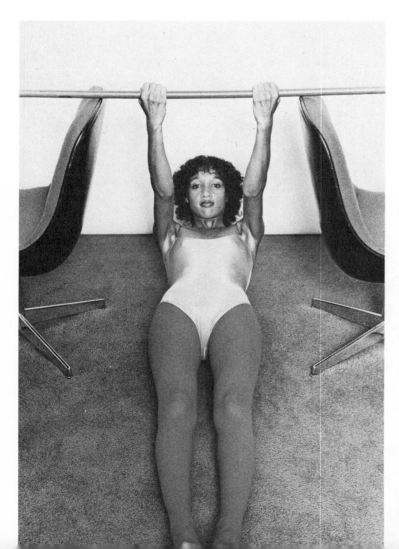
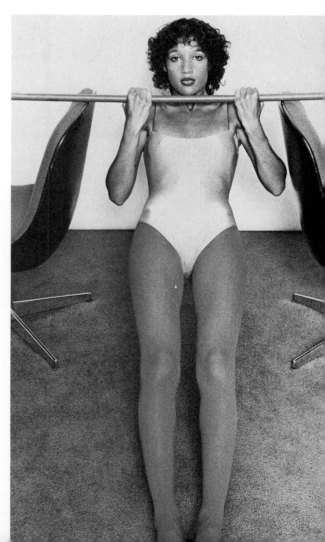

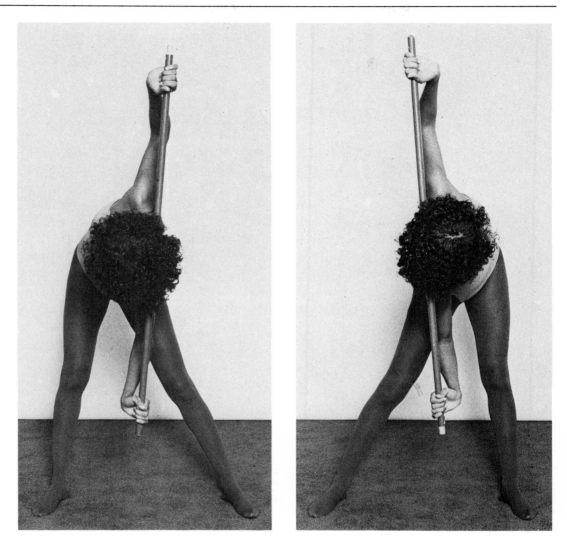

TWISTS WITH A BROOMSTICK

PURPOSE: To slim the waistline.

Stand with your legs spread wide and your back straight. Hold a broomstick behind your neck, gripping it wide with both hands. Bend at the waist and twist your body in a half-circular motion. In the extreme position, the broomstick should point at the floor. Note: It is important to use the full motion in this exercise.

Alternate left, right, left, right.

BREATHING: Should be rhythmical—in with one full twist, out with the next full twist.

REPS: 10 to each side, working up to 30 to each side

SETS: 2

LATERAL RAISES

PURPOSE: To firm and shape the shoulders.

Take a dumbbell in each hand and stand with your arms at your sides, palms facing your thighs. Without bending your arms, slowly raise the dumbbells out and up as far as you can. Pause. Then slowly let them return to the beginning position. Do not allow your arms to rotate (in the extreme position, your palms should be facing the floor).

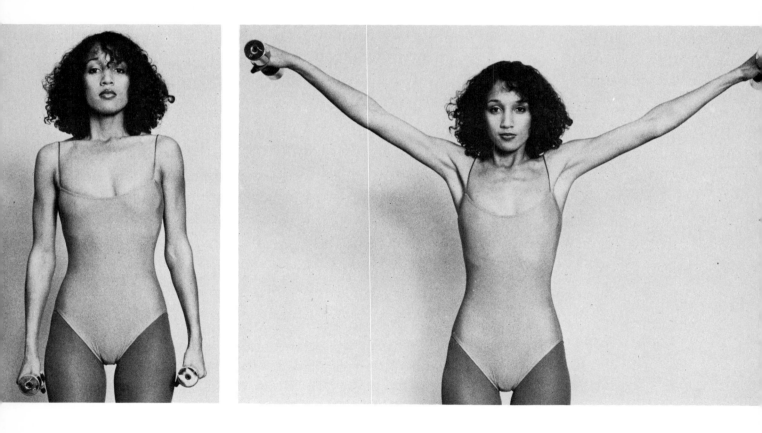

BREATHING:	Exhale as you lift; inhale as you lower it.
WEIGHT:	3–5 pounds
REPS:	10
SETS:	2, increasing to 3 in the fourth week

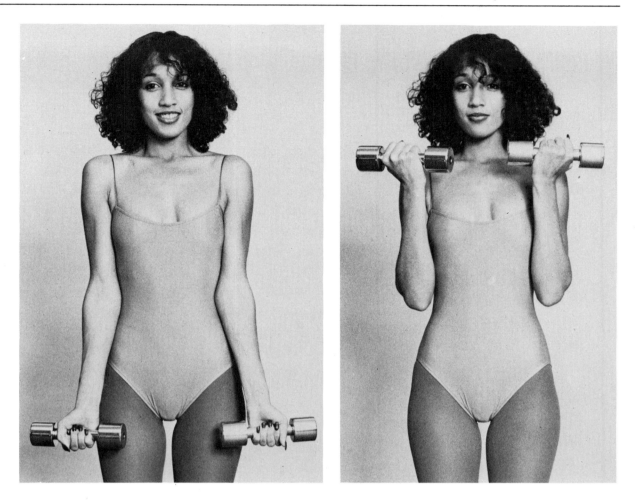

DUMBBELL CURLS

PURPOSE: To tone and strengthen the biceps.

Stand with a dumbbell in each hand, palms facing outward.
Press your upper arms against your side and lift the weights, moving
only your forearms. In the extreme position, the weights should touch
the top of your chest.

Slowly let the weight back to your thighs.

BREATHING: Exhale as you lift; inhale as you lower weight.
WEIGHT: 3–5 pounds
REPS: 10
SETS: 2, increasing to 3 in the fourth week

SERIES 2
Gymwork

GOOD GYMS are designed to provide the proper equipment to train your body in the most effective way. Going to a gym is like going to a specialist. There are machines for every part of the body. Most of the machines utilize weight to create resistance, and most are built specifically for one muscle group. Machines have the great advantage of allowing you to concentrate on working the muscle and not on balancing the weight at the same time. This isolates the muscle and makes the work 100 percent effective.

There are a number of good reasons for choosing one gym over another. Obviously, one of these is location. It should be convenient. It should also be progressive—in looks and in the attitude of the people who run it. I have not called for exercises that require exotic or special machines, mainly because I believe in the effectiveness of basic, straightforward movements. However, the equipment in the gym you choose ought to be up-to-date and extensive enough to fulfill your needs. The exercise rooms should be well lighted, well ventilated, and roomy enough to allow you to work out in comfort. The showers and locker rooms should be clean and spacious. Most important: You should feel good—energized and enthusiastic—when you are there.

Try to work out at the gym with a friend. Companionship is important, especially if you are the kind of person who needs encouragement and challenge. A friend should be helpful, someone who can watch you and offer constructive criticism as well as support. By observing and helping each other, you can recognize and correct your own mistakes more easily.

Finally, the one thing that will make your program totally successful is your attitude.

Note: Fewer repetitions with more weight result in building size and mass. More repetitions with less weight result in a decrease of the size of a particular body part.

OUTER THIGH CABLE PULLS

PURPOSE: To trim the outer thighs.

This exercise focuses mainly on the muscles in the outer portion of the thigh, an area where many women put on fat and often develop what are called saddlebags.

For this exercise, use a cable machine in the high pulley station, with 10 pounds of weight. Lie on the floor, supporting yourself on your elbows. Place your body perpendicular to the base of the machine, with the collar around your right ankle. Bend your left leg at the knee. Begin with your right leg straight in the air and push it outward until your toes point away from the machine. Do not allow

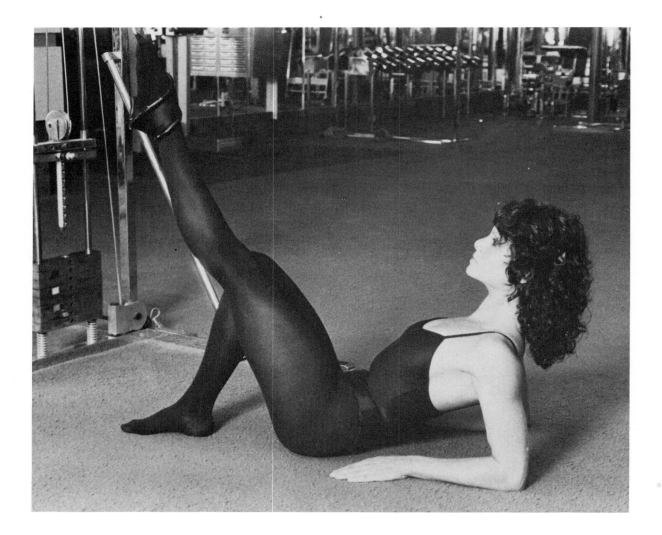

either your bent leg or your pelvis to move. If you begin to roll, brace yourself better.

Move your leg as fast as you can and still keep your body and the machine under complete control. Speed is important, but if you move your leg too fast, the cable may go slack and give jerky resistance, which lessens its effect on your muscles. The ideal thing is to set a pace that is smooth but demanding. Do a large number of repetitions and really burn off the fat. Increase the number as you can, without sacrificing the smooth rhythmical movement.

BREATHING: Exhale as you push your leg to the extreme position away from the machine; inhale as you let it back.
WEIGHT: 10 pounds
REPS: 40 with each leg
SETS: 2, increasing to 3 in the second week

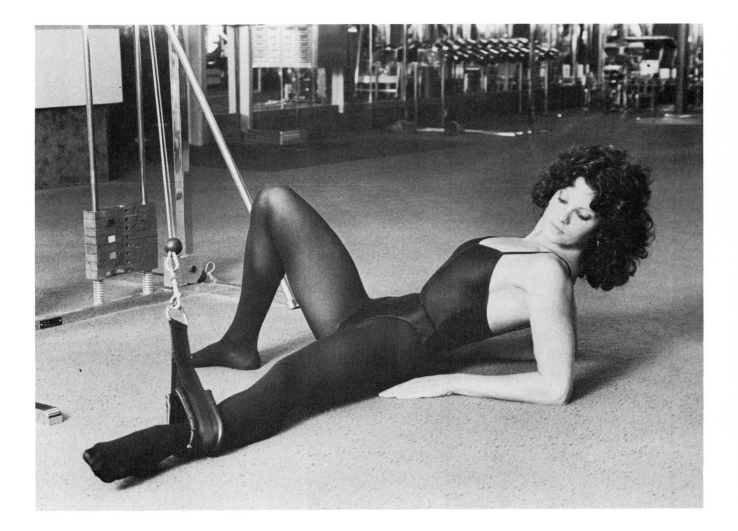

INNER THIGH CABLE PULLS

PURPOSE: To tone and smooth the inner thighs.

Lie on the floor with your head facing the cable machine. Rest your weight on your hands and elbows. Attach the ankle collar, with the cable running to the high pulley station, to your right ankle. Then, keeping your left leg slightly bent on the floor and your right leg straight, lower your right leg. Work for a maximum range of

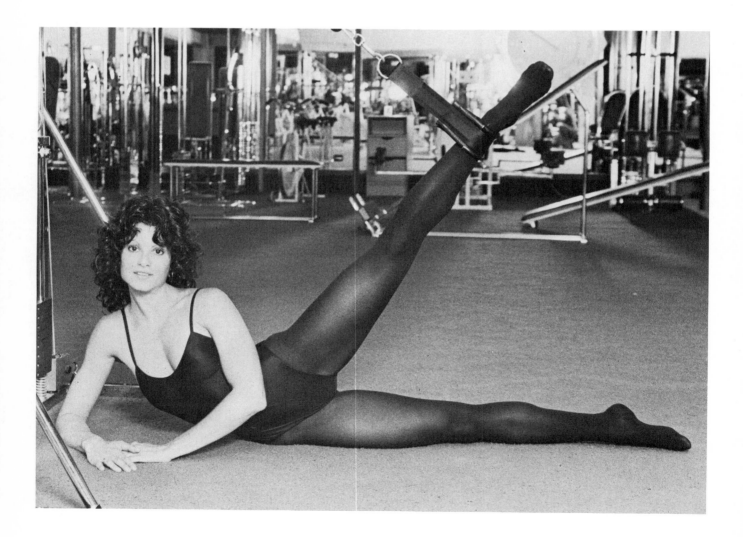

movement. As you lift your leg, you will feel the muscles stretching; and as you lower it back to the floor, you will feel them contracting.

One thing to watch in this exercise is to make sure your knee points straight ahead. If the knee is allowed to rotate, you will work the rear thigh muscles instead of the inner thigh muscles.

BREATHING: Exhale as you lift your leg; inhale as you lower it.
WEIGHT: 10 pounds, increase as needed
REPS: 20 each leg, increasing to 40. Note: If you need to build up your legs, do fewer repetitions with more weight.
SETS: 2, increasing to 3 in the third week

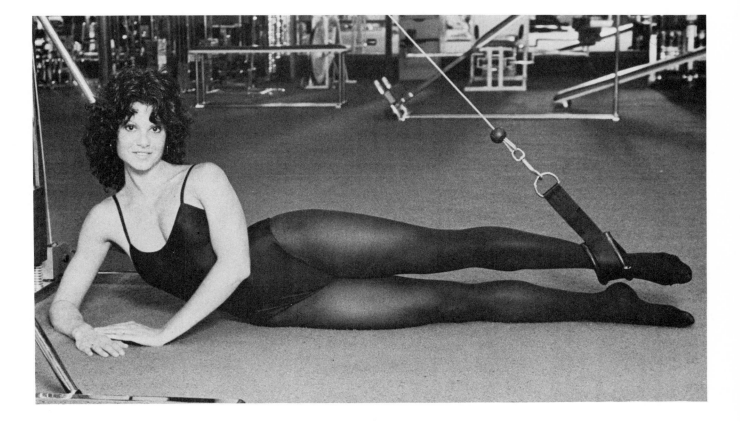

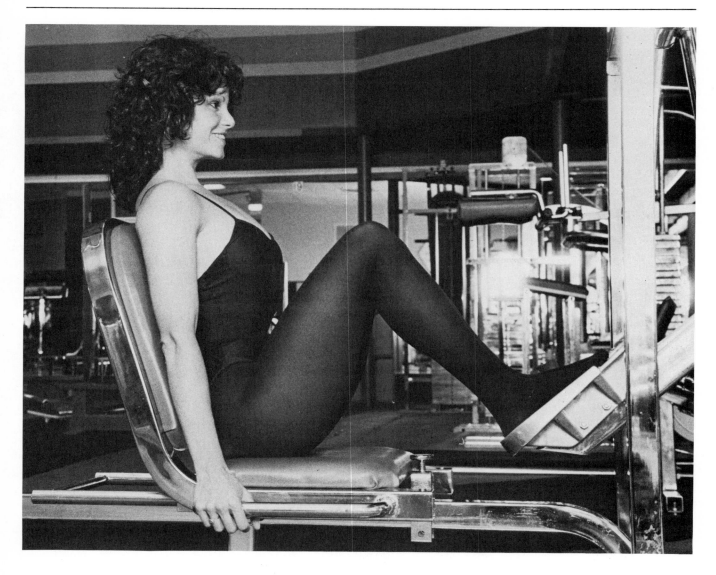

LEG PRESS ON A MACHINE

PURPOSE: To trim and tighten, or to increase the buttocks.

Get on the leg press machine, with your feet situated a few inches apart on the pedals and your knees bent.

In a smooth, rhythmical motion, push against the pedals until your knees are locked straight, as you see in the photographs. Then let them return slowly to a bent position. You will be working two muscle groups. The main group is the buttocks, and the other one is on the front of the thigh near the knee. Both of these muscles are contracting to straighten the leg against the resistance of the weight.

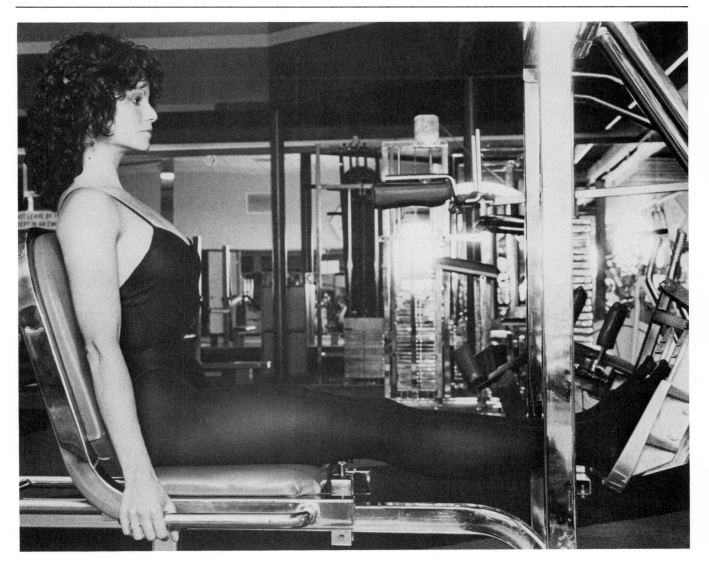

To lose fat from your buttocks and thighs, do the leg presses with a light weight and a high number of repetitions.

To build thighs that are too thin or to fill out your buttocks, add more weight and do fewer repetitions.

BREATHING: Exhale as you push; inhale as you let your legs return to beginning position.
WEIGHT: 10–20 pounds
REPS: 20, increasing to 50
SETS: 2

LEG EXTENSIONS

PURPOSE: To tone and maintain the frontal thighs, especially the lower frontal thighs.

Sit on the leg extension machine so your knees just bend over the edge of the bench. Hook your toes under the bar and grasp the sides of the bench slightly behind you as a brace, but keep your back straight.

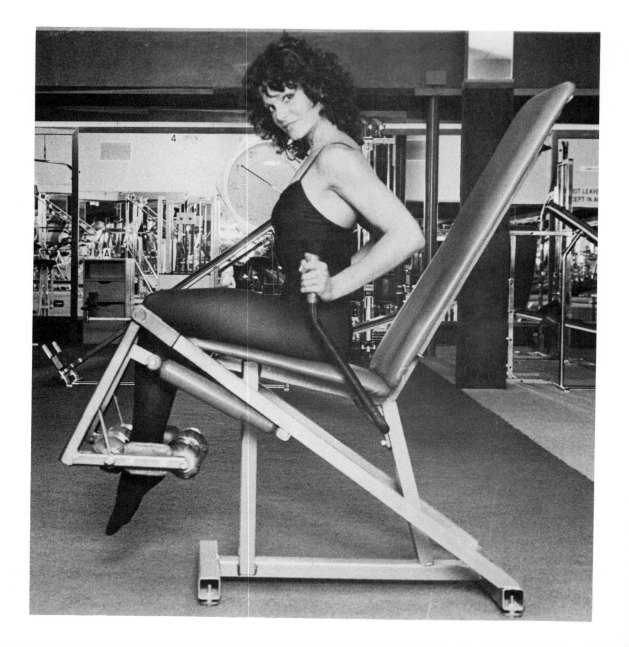

Using a smooth, steady motion, push the bar up until your legs are straight. Hold this position for a few seconds; then begin lowering your legs at the same controlled rate of speed, allowing your muscles to work against the resistance, and let the bar come back down.

There is really no better exercise than leg extensions to firm the frontal thigh muscles.

BREATHING: Exhale as you lift weight; inhale as you lower it.
WEIGHT: 20 pounds
REPS: 12
SETS: 2, increasing to 3 in the third week

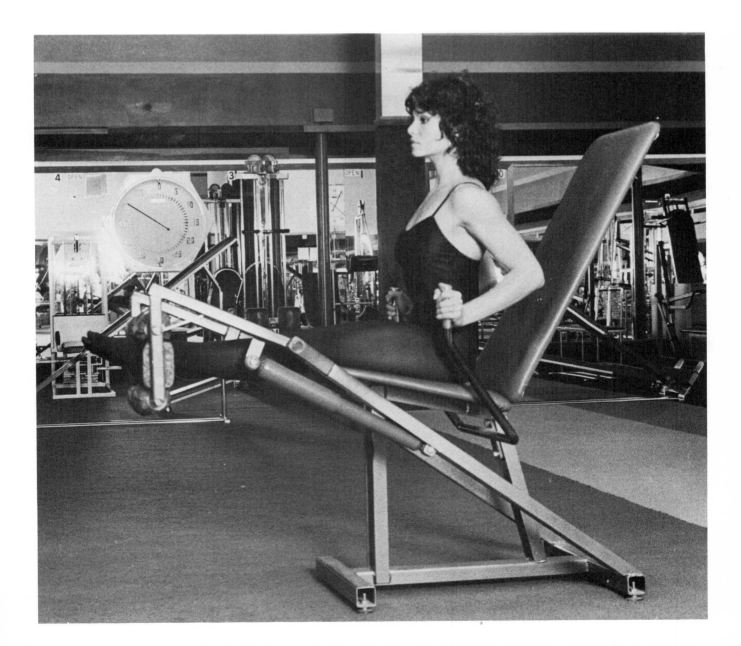

CALF RAISES ON A MACHINE

PURPOSE: To build and maintain the calves.

Many women want to increase the size of their calves in order to make their bodies more symmetrical. The simplest way to do it is on a multipress machine, although if that is not available in your particular gym, it can also be done on a 2-inch wood block with a barbell held across your shoulders. Your toes should be elevated on a block of wood so a full stretch is obtained when your heel is fully lifted off the floor.

With the weight on your shoulders, lift your heels up as high as you can; then lower them to the floor. This full movement contracts the muscles of the calf, giving it a round, definite shape.

BREATHING: Exhale as you lift onto tiptoe; inhale as you let yourself back down.
WEIGHT: 50 pounds
REPS: 10
SETS: 5

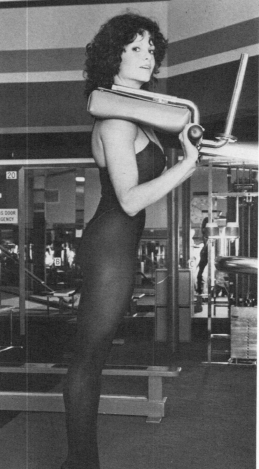

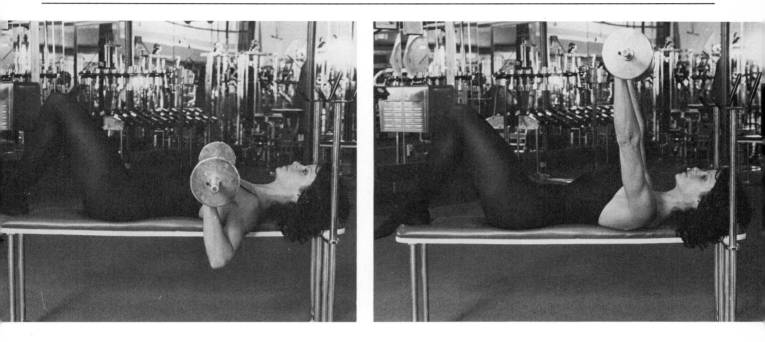

BENCH PRESS

PURPOSE: To firm and strengthen the pectoral muscles.

Well-developed pectorals can give even a small-breasted woman the look of cleavage. They act as supporting fingers to hold up the breasts, whatever their size, and make them look more beautiful by expanding the breastplate.

Lie on the exercise bench with your legs bent and ankles crossed. Gripping the barbell from 28 to 30 inches wide, balance it just above your chest.

Push the barbell overhead, lock your elbows in the extreme position, pause, then let the barbell down slowly to beginning position. You may not be able to do 5 repetitions at first, so try doing fewer repetitions and more sets. Increase the number of repetitions as you become stronger.

BREATHING: Inhale while lowering the barbell; exhale while pressing it up.
WEIGHT: 30–50 pounds
REPS: 5, increasing to 10
SETS: 4, increasing to 6 in the third week

FRONT PRESS WITH BARBELL

PURPOSE: To smooth and tone the shoulders and the backs of the arms.

Many women have bony shoulders. The front press with a barbell will develop the front deltoid muscle and help eliminate that problem.

Begin with your feet approximately a foot apart, grip the barbell —with your palms down—and lift it to your chest in a single movement (this is called "cleaning the weight" in bodybuilding). Then press it slowly and smoothly over your head and lock your elbows.

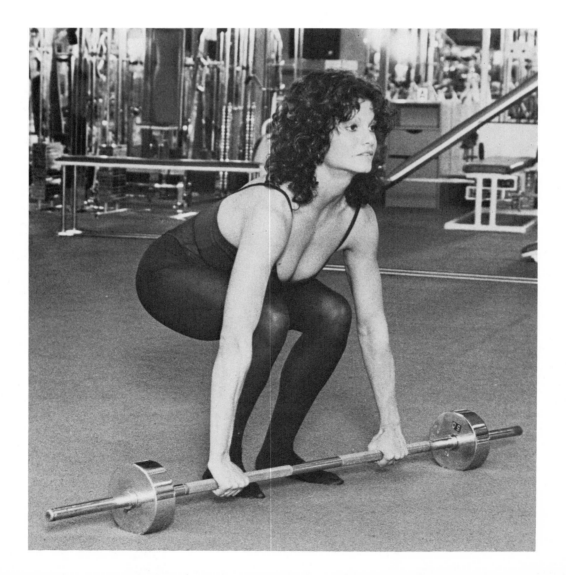

Study the photographs carefully and follow the steps as I have outlined them. Once you have mastered the movements and are doing the press in the proper form, you can add more weight.

BREATHING: Exhale as you lift; inhale as you lower the weight.
WEIGHT: 20 pounds
REPS: 10
SETS: 2, increasing to 3 in the third week

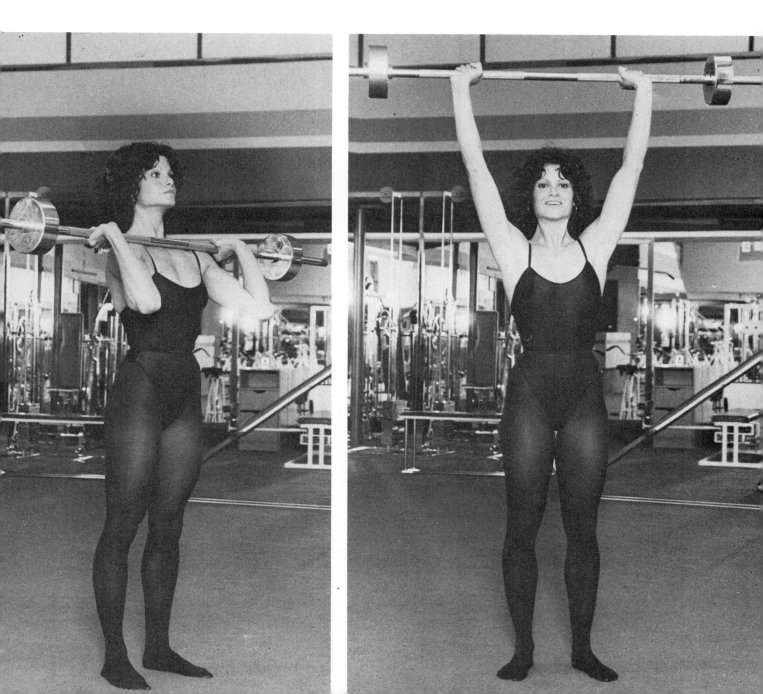

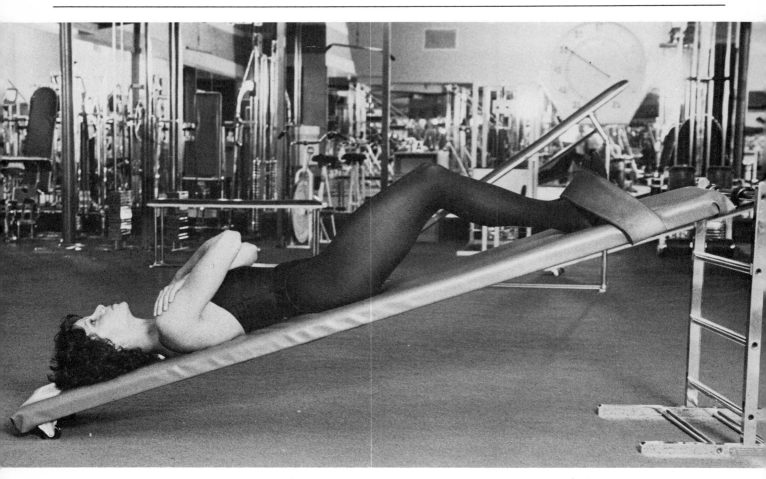

BENT-KNEE SIT-UPS

PURPOSE: To tighten the upper abdominals.

Bent-knee sit-ups give you the kind of flat, firm stomach that looks fantastic in a bikini.

Lie down on a slant board, hook your ankles under the rollers or strap, and crisscross your arms across your chest with the palms on your shoulders (crossed arms eliminate any assistance from your arms).

Pull your body up about a third of the way, and then make sure you go back down far enough to touch the vertebrae at your waistline.

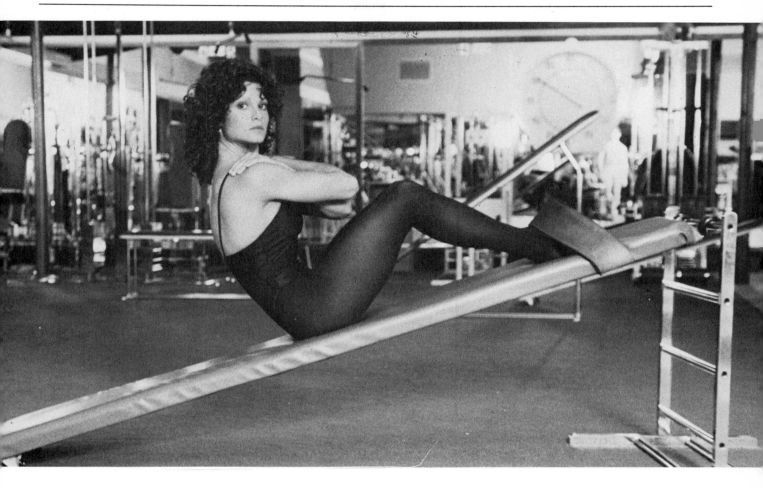

For a really flat, firm stomach, do the movements slowly, with absolutely no jerking. Remember to hold in your stomach as you do this exercise to increase the amount of contraction. As with crunches, contracting the abdominal muscles is what tightens and flattens the stomach. In this exercise, it is not necessary to make a full range of the movement.

BREATHING: Exhale as you pull your body up; inhale as you let it back.
REPS: 10, increasing to 50
SETS: 2, increasing to 3

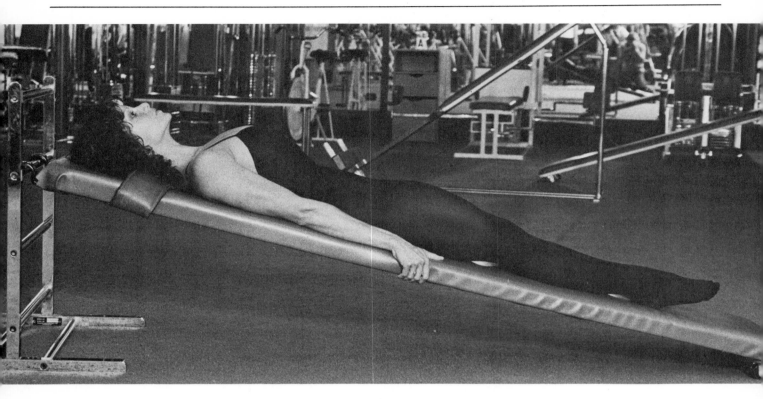

ALTERNATE LEG RAISES

PURPOSE: To firm and flatten the lower abdominal muscles.

Some women have a small waist and trim hips, but have developed a pouchy lower stomach. This can easily be corrected by doing these bent and straight leg raises. These exercises are done on an exercise board or on the floor.

Lie on your back with your head raised high enough so you can tuck your chin into your chest. Flatten your hands, palms down, under your buttocks.

Pull your knees up toward your chest and then return them to the legs-straight-out starting position.

In the second movement, hold your legs straight and lift them as high in the air as you can; then lower them back to the starting position.

BREATHING: Exhale as you lift your legs; inhale as you lower them.
REPS: 25, increasing to 50
SETS: 2, increasing to 3 in the third week

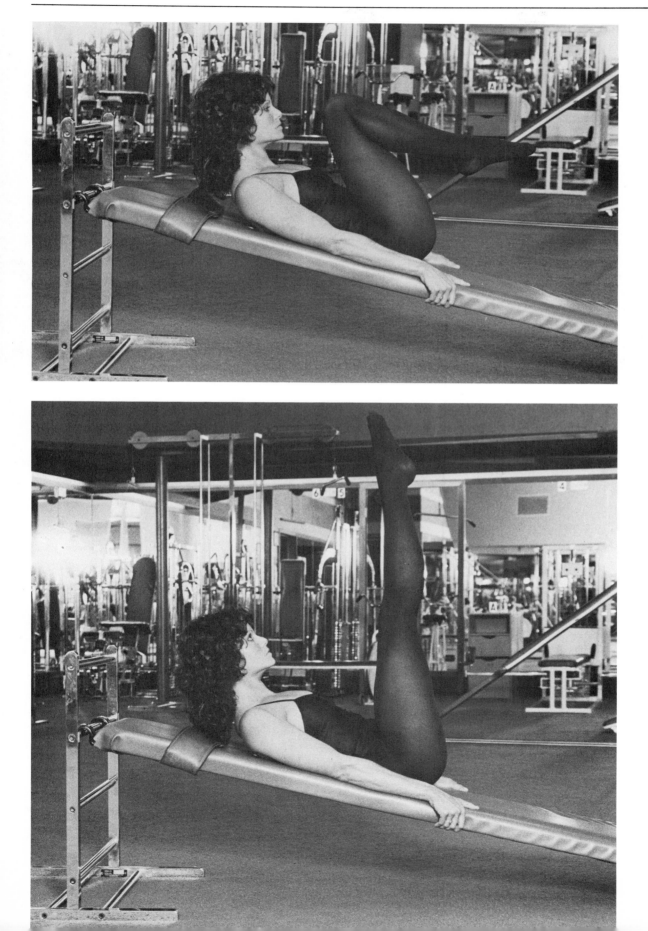

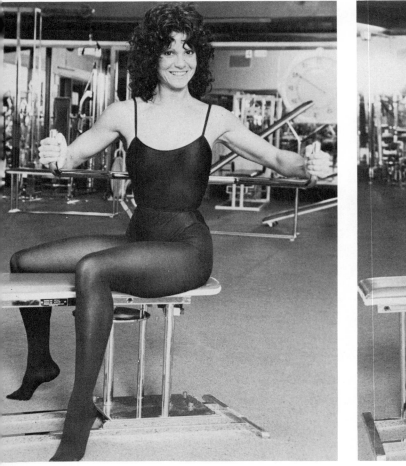 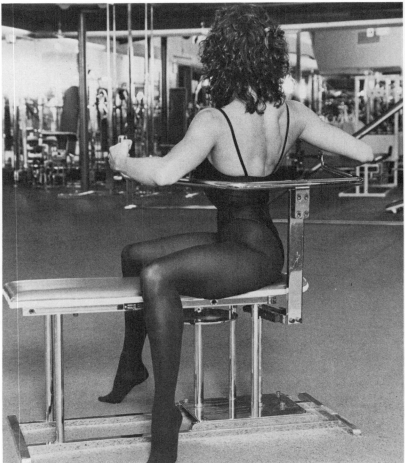

TWISTS ON A MACHINE

PURPOSE: To trim the waist.

The first exercise works the oblique muscles in the upper part of your waist. Sit on the twister bench and grasp the arm bars. Keep your pelvis still and move your torso from side to side.

The second oblique exercise works your lower waist. Step onto the free-moving disk of the twist machine and take a firm hold on the stationary bar. Now spin your pelvis from side to side, keeping your upper body static. The movement here should all be from the waist down.

BREATHING: Rhythmical
REPS: Because these exercises are done rapidly, it is easier to
              measure them in minutes rather than reps: 3 minutes,
              increasing 1 minute per week to 5 minutes.

Note: Twists will thoroughly exercise your obliques and trim your
waistline. If you have excess fat in your midriff section, you should
concentrate mainly on the seated twist exercise. If you tend to be
heavier in the stomach, you should work harder on the standing twists.

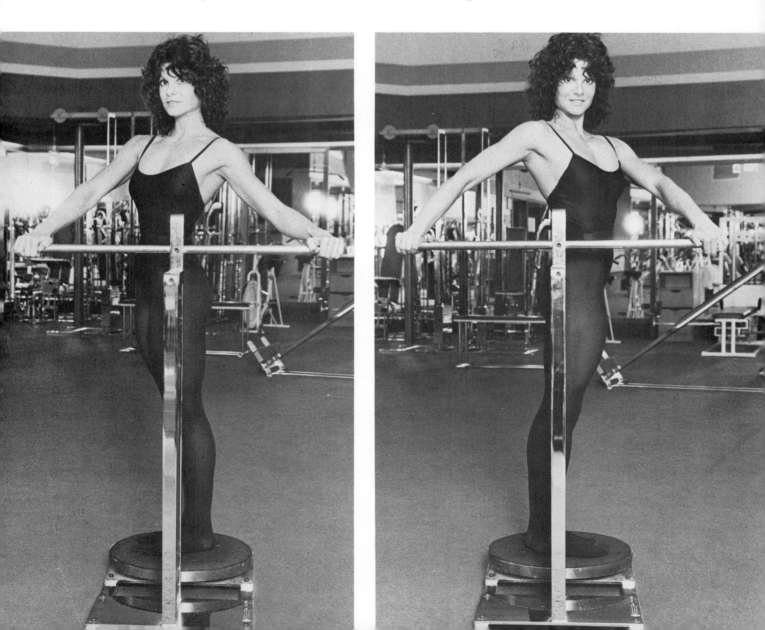

REVERSE CURLS

PURPOSE: To strengthen and develop the forearms and hands.

Grasp the barbell with your palms facing down. Lift the barbell to chest level—palms facing away from you—and let it down again.

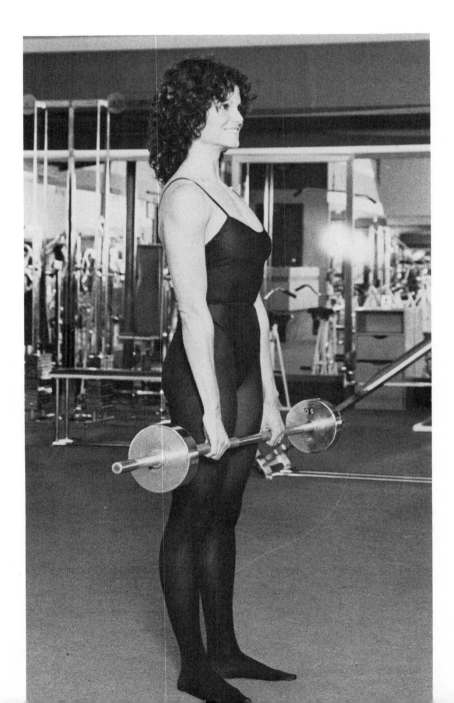

BREATHING: Exhale as you lift bar; inhale as you lower it.
WEIGHT: 10 pounds, increase to 20
REPS: 10
SETS: 2, increasing to 3 in the third week

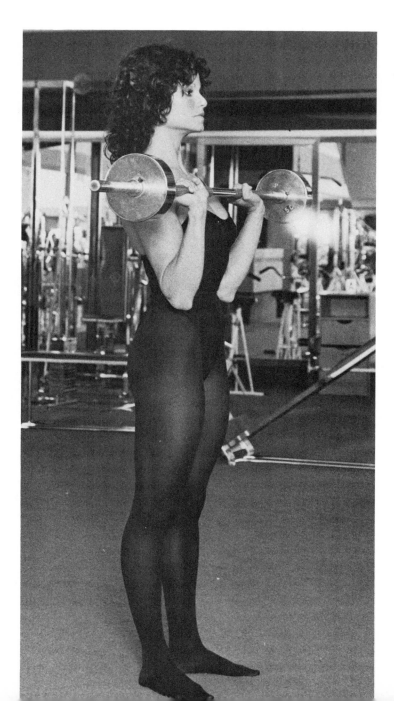

SERIES 3
The Supersets

A SUPERSET is two exercises for related or complementary muscles or muscle groups—biceps and triceps, back and chest—with no rest interval between them. It is an advanced program for anyone serious about the ultimate in exercise. The superset series is designed to:

- *Save time by cutting out rest periods*
- *Further strengthen your cardiovascular system by keeping blood flowing from one area to another*
- *Increase the oxygenation of your blood*
- *Enable you to burn off more fat*

Note: Fewer repetitions with more weight result in building size and mass. More repetitions with less weight result in a decrease of the size of a particular body part.

SUPERSET 1

TWO-PART LEG RAISES

PURPOSE: To flatten and reduce the stomach.

      Sit on the edge of a high bench and lean back until you are resting on your hands.

      Bring your knees up until they touch your chest, then push them to the floor again. (This exercise loses effectiveness if you change the position of your torso, so do not lie back while you are pulling up your knees.)

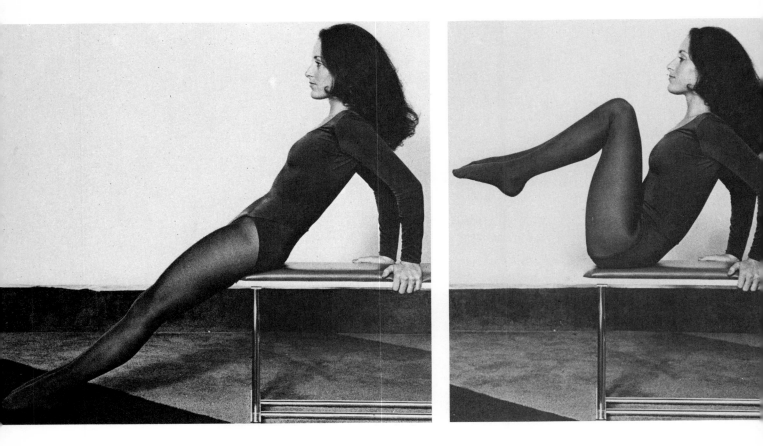

Now, keeping your legs straight, lift them as far as possible, pause, then lower them back to the starting position.

BREATHING: Exhale as you bring your legs up; inhale as you let them down.
REPS: 10, increasing to 20
SETS: 2, increasing to 3 in the third week.

Without resting, go immediately to the Cable Bends to the Side to superset all the muscles in your waistline.

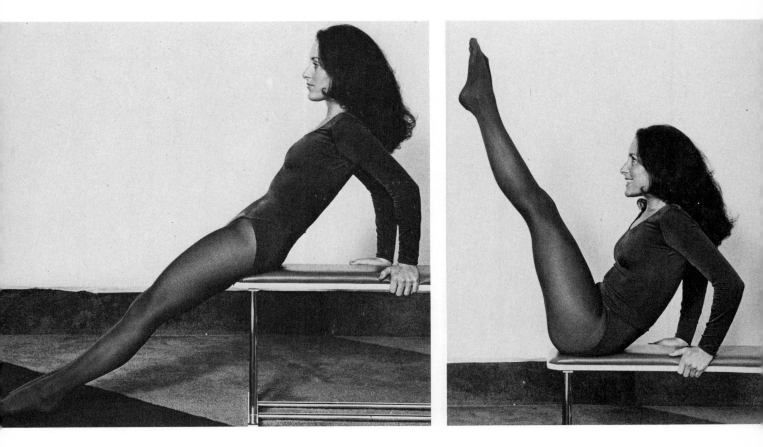

SIDE BENDS WITH A CABLE

PURPOSE: To trim the waist.

Do this exercise on a cable machine with the hand-pull attached to the low pulley station. Stand with your left side toward the machine and place your legs about 2 feet apart. Make sure you are far enough away from the machine so the weights will not come to rest when you lean to the left. Hold the handle of the cable with your left hand and place your right hand behind your neck, to help keep your posture correct during the movements.

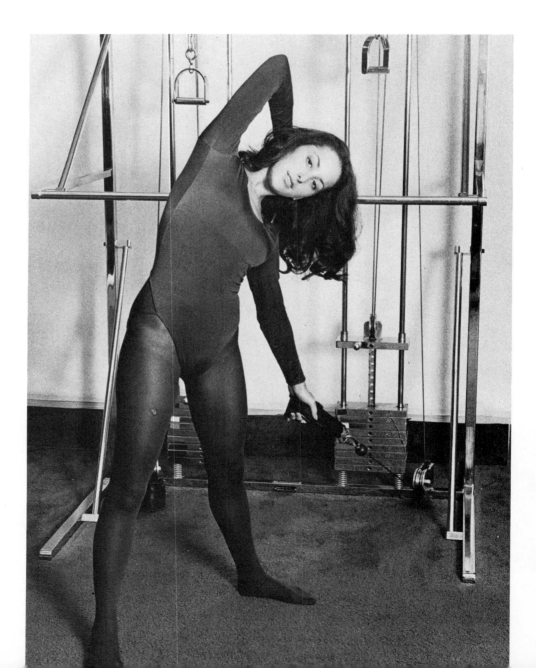

Maintaining a perfect upright position, lean first toward the machine, then away from it, dropping your right shoulder as low as possible.

Turn and take the cable with your right hand. Repeat the movements.

BREATHING: Exhale as you lean toward the machine; inhale as you lean away.
WEIGHT: 10 pounds
REPS: 25 to each side
SETS: 2, increasing to 3 in the third week

Rest one minute before starting the next superset.

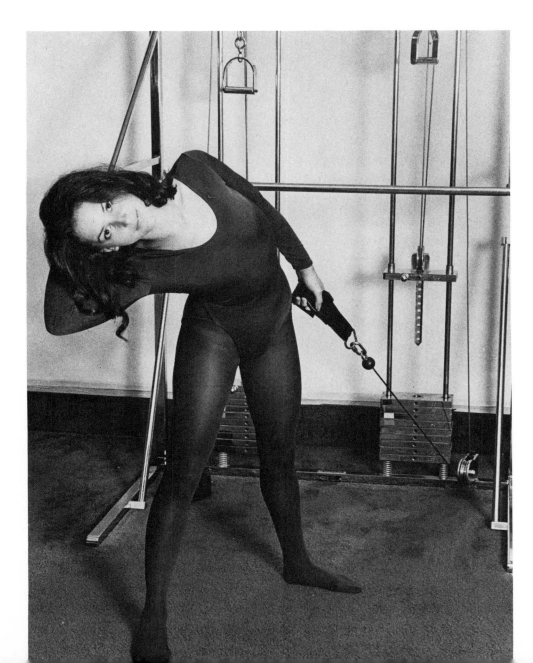

SUPERSET 2

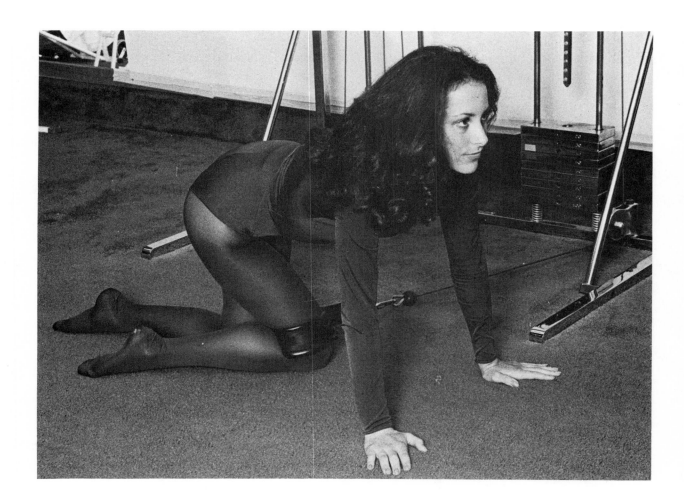

KNEELING CABLE PULLS

PURPOSE: To reduce, tone, and smooth the outer thigh.

This exercise is also done on the cable machine in the low pulley station. It might seem awkward at first, but once you're in position, you'll find it's not that difficult.

Get on hands and knees parallel to the machine. Take the collar that is normally attached to your ankle and fasten it near the knee on your right leg, which should be farthest from the machine. Your right leg will be pulled in front of your left leg as the weight draws it toward the machine.

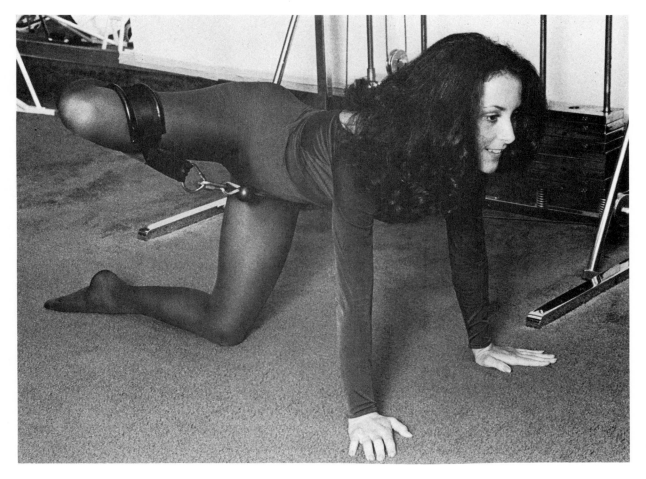

Now pull your leg away from the machine, keeping your knee bent and lifting it as high as possible. Your legs should be at right angles to each other—as you see in the photograph.

Change positions on the floor and attach the cable to your left leg.

BREATHING: Exhale as you pull your leg away from the machine; inhale as you let it return toward the machine.

WEIGHT: 10 pounds
REPS: 20, increasing to 40
SETS: 2, increasing to 3 in the third week

Go immediately to the sitting cable pulls. These two exercises, done in conjunction, will work the entire thigh area and help to emphasize the soft flowing lines of the upper leg.

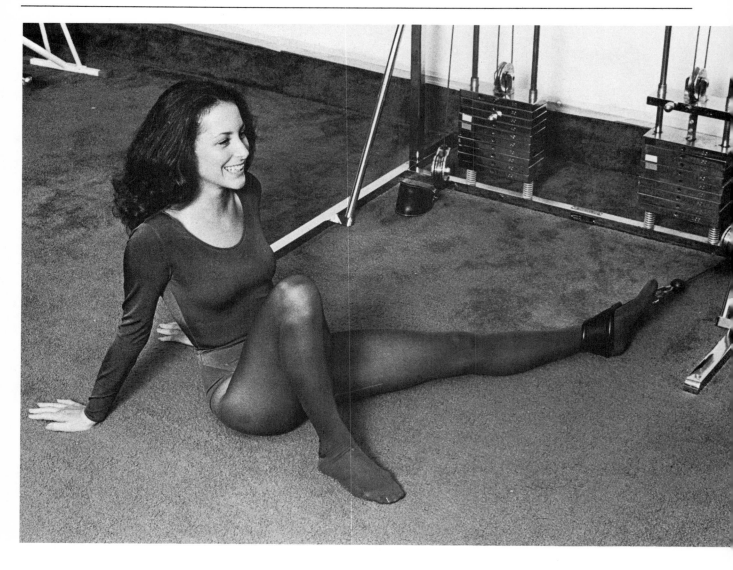

SITTING CABLE PULLS

PURPOSE: To reduce and firm the inner thighs.

Sitting with your left side toward the cable machine, attach the low pulley collar to your left ankle. Lean back slightly and rest on your hands for support. Your right leg should be bent at the knee. It can either rest on the floor so the leg is flat or point in the air, whichever position is most comfortable.

Point the toe of your left leg and allow the weight to pull it toward the machine; then bring it back until it is straight in front of

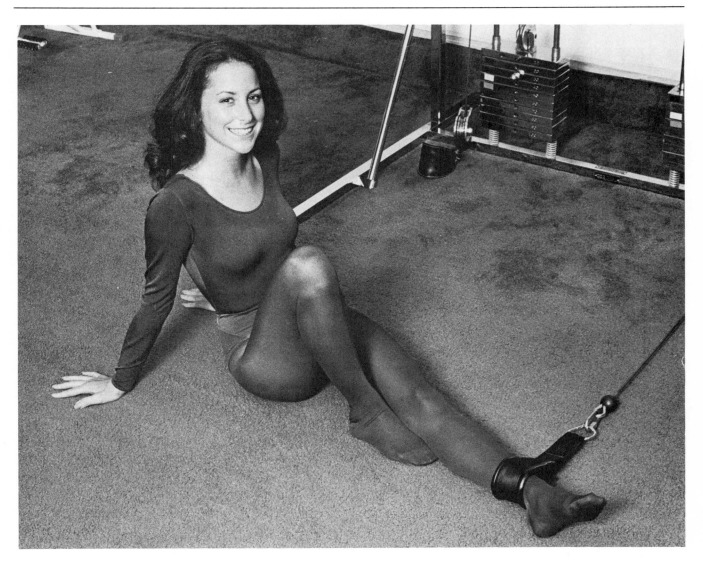

your body. You must point your toe during the movement in order to isolate the inner thigh muscles.

Reverse your position and attach the cable to your right ankle.

BREATHING: Exhale as you pull your leg away from the machine; inhale as you let it move toward the machine.
WEIGHT: 10 pounds
REPS: 25, increasing to 40 for each leg
SETS: 2, increasing to 3 in the third week

Relax for a minute before beginning the next routine.

SUPERSET 3

PARALLEL SQUATS

PURPOSE: To firm the buttocks and reduce the front of the thighs.

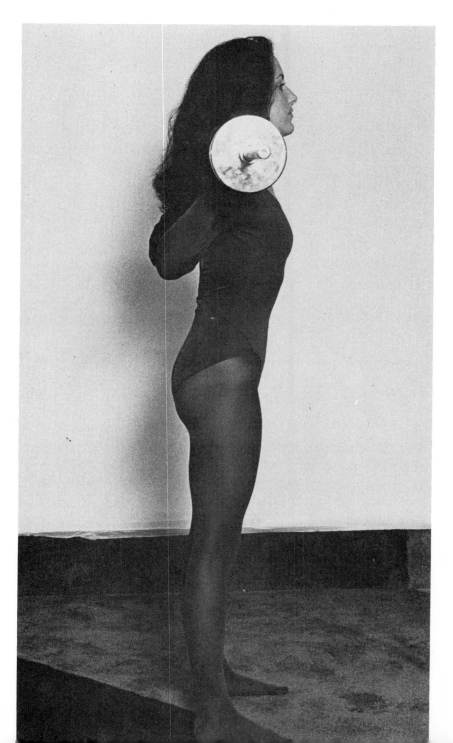

Because of the effort required, squats will strengthen your heart and lungs and improve your circulation. They are especially helpful in conditioning yourself for skiing, biking, running, tennis.

Balance a barbell behind your neck. Keep your upper body straight and lower yourself down into a squat position, until your thighs are parallel to the floor.

Do the squat in front of a mirror so you can check your form. Don't squat lower than a position parallel to the floor because this could be harmful to anyone with weak knees.

BREATHING: Inhale on the way down; exhale while coming up.
WEIGHT: 20 pounds, increasing to 40
REPS: 8
SETS: 2, increasing to 3 in the third week

Without resting, move to the Leg Curls on a Machine to complete the superset for your legs.

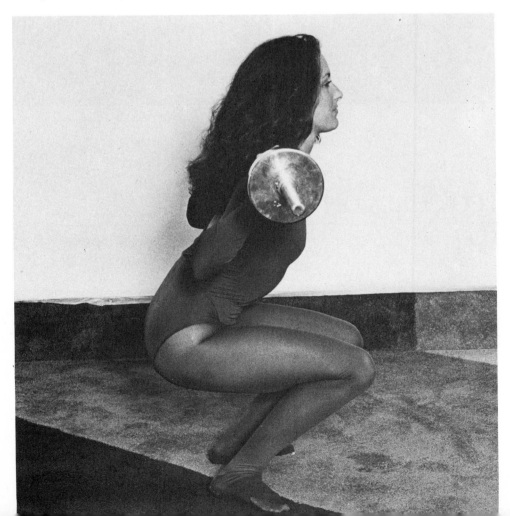

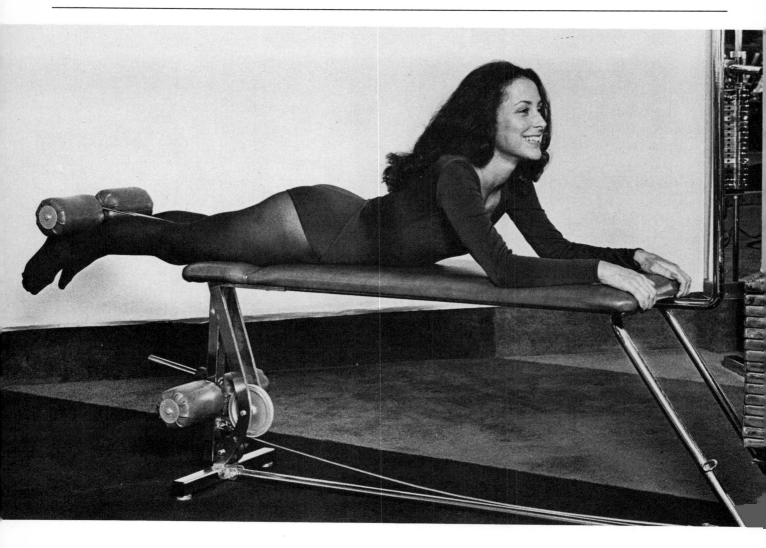

LEG CURLS ON A MACHINE

PURPOSE: To reduce and tone muscles in back of the upper leg.

Lie on your stomach on the bench of the leg curl machine. Hook your heels under the lever bar. Then, holding the sides of the bench firmly with your hands, pull the bar toward your buttocks. Bring your heels as far forward as you can; then let the weight back down slowly. Be sure to allow the bar to return all the way so your leg

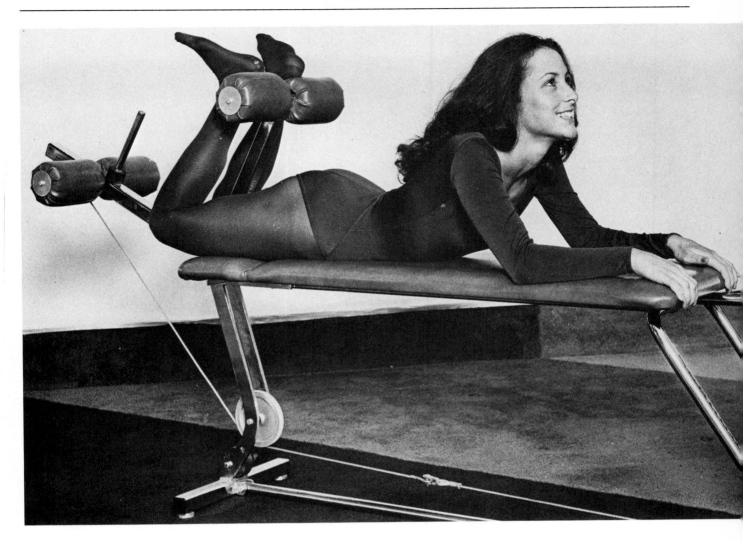

muscles get fully stretched. The proper form, which will give you the most direct and immediate results, is to move your leg only from the knee down.

BREATHING: Exhale as you lift; inhale as you lower weight.
WEIGHT: 10 pounds
REPS: 10, increasing to 30
SETS: 2, increasing to 3 in the third week

Rest for one minute.

SUPERSET 4

NARROW GRIP PULLDOWN

PURPOSE: To tone back muscles and shape up the upper arms.

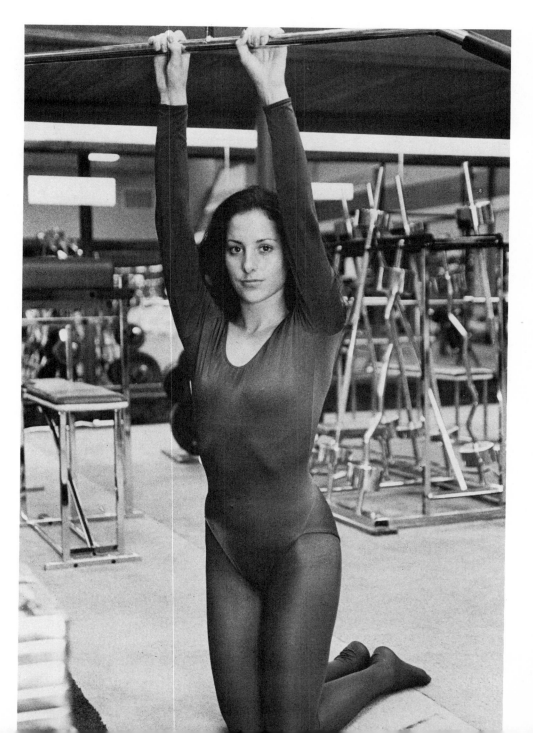

Sit on the bench facing the pulldown machine. Gripping the bar just slightly narrower than shoulder width, pull it down to chest level. Be sure to use a smooth, steady motion.

Let the bar return slowly to the up position, making full use of the negative force. Keep your back straight and allow your arms to go up until you feel the stretch in your back and arms.

BREATHING: Exhale as you pull down; inhale as you let bar go up.
WEIGHT: 20 pounds
REPS: 10–12
SETS: 2, increasing to 3 in the third week

Go on to the Dumbbell Flys, which will complete the work on your upper back and chest muscles.

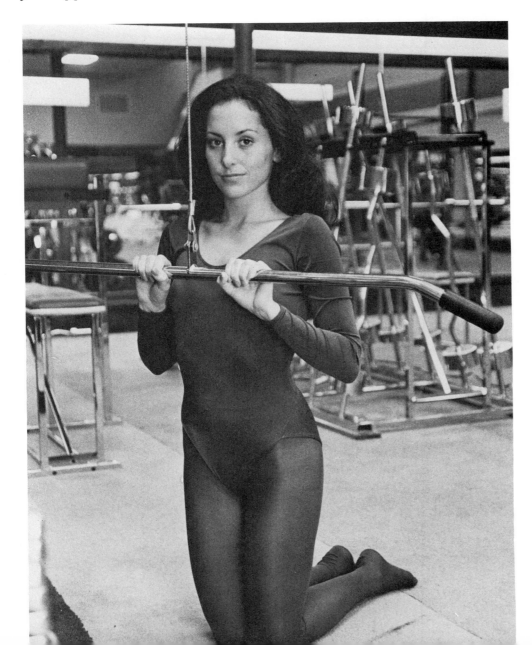

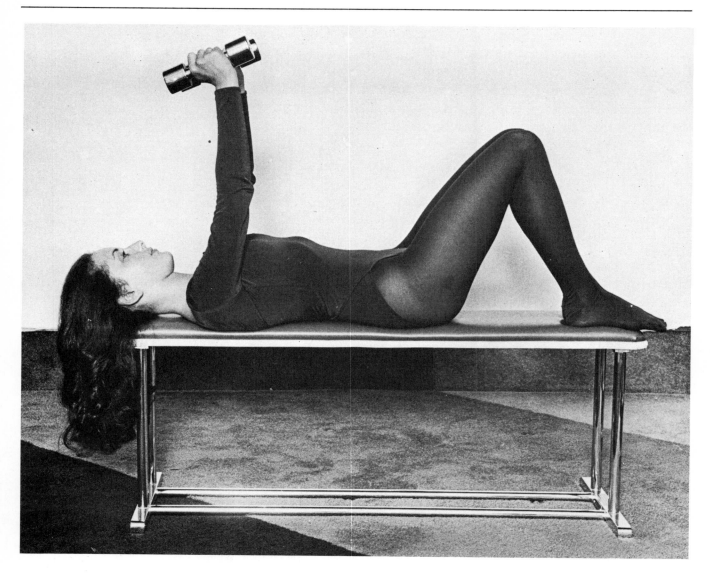

DUMBBELL FLYS

PURPOSE: To firm and build the muscles constituting the bustline.

    Take a dumbbell in each hand and lie on your back on an exercise bench. The movement is like a flying motion with your arms going from the top position, straight above the chest, down as close to the floor as they can reach.

    By keeping your arms straight and your knees bent while lying on the bench, you work the pectoral muscles with no assistance from

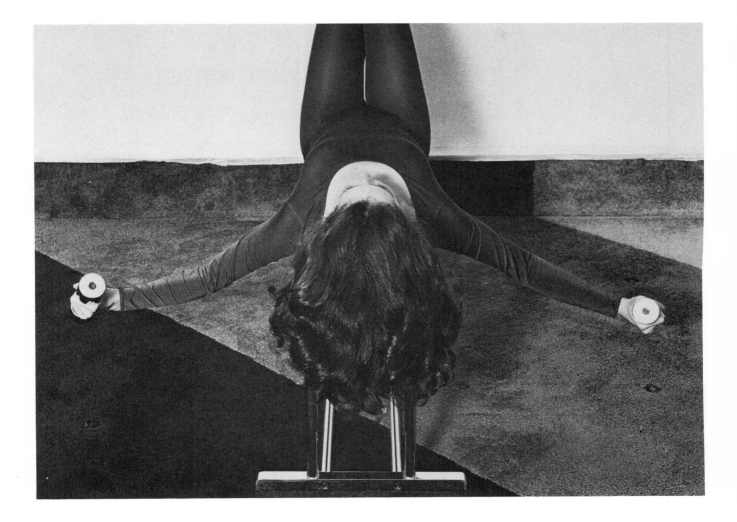

the abdominals. The number of repetitions is more important than the amount of weight.

BREATHING: Exhale as you bring the dumbbells above your chest; inhale as you lower them.

WEIGHT: 3 pounds in each hand, increasing to 5

REPS: 10, increasing to 20

SETS: 2, increasing to 3 in the third week

Relax with your arms loosely at your sides for one minute before going to the next superset.

SUPERSET 5

SIDE LATERALS WITH DUMBBELLS

PURPOSE: To reduce and beautify the shoulders.

This exercise works the muscles in the shoulder, known as the side deltoids, and helps create a very smooth, good-looking upper torso, especially in the area where the arm joins the body.

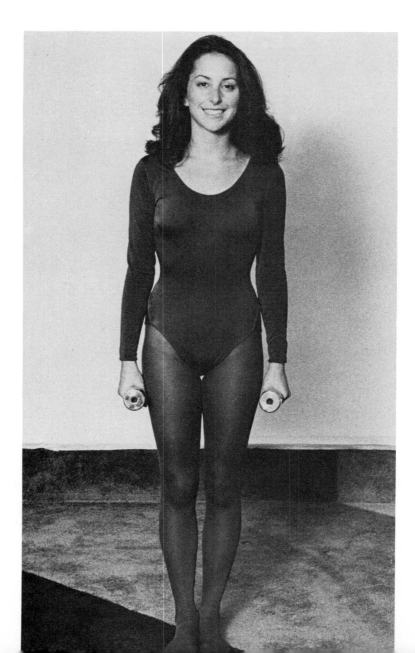

Stand with your feet together. Take one lightweight dumbbell in each hand and hold them at your sides.

Lift your arms straight out to at least shoulder level, without bending your elbows, and then let them back down again.

BREATHING: Exhale as you lift the dumbbells; inhale as you let them return to your sides.
WEIGHT: 3 pounds, increasing to 5
REPS: 10, increasing to 25
SETS: 2, increasing to 3 in the third week

Go immediately to the Upper Arm Extensions.

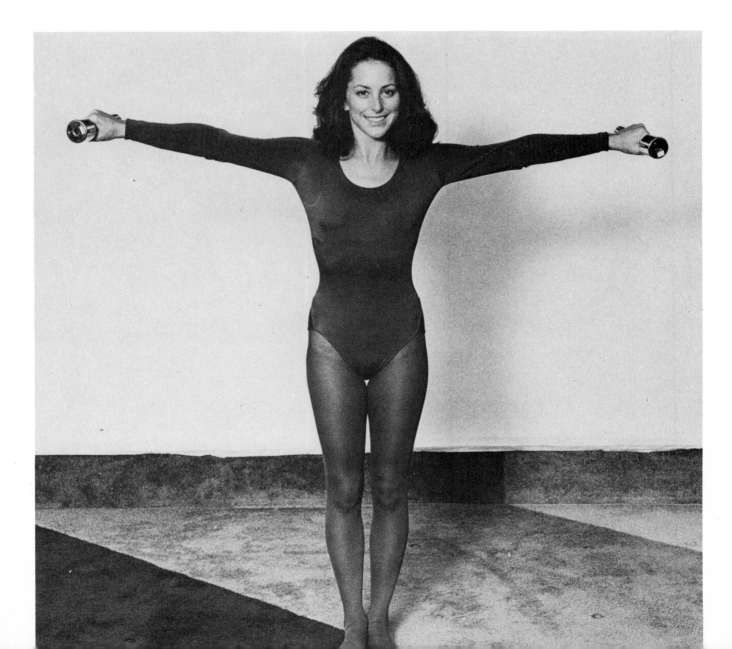

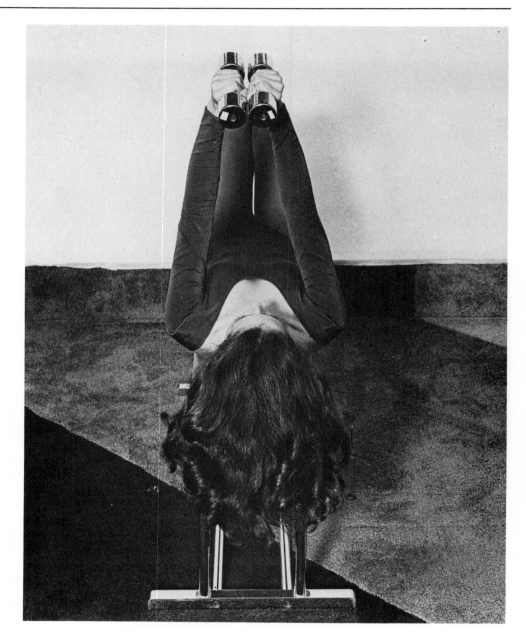

UPPER ARM EXTENSIONS

PURPOSE: To reduce and tighten the back of the upper arm.

The time when I notice a woman's triceps is almost invariably when she's pointing or gesturing. What I often *see* is not flattering: It's a flabby, unused muscle hanging down from the backs of her arms.

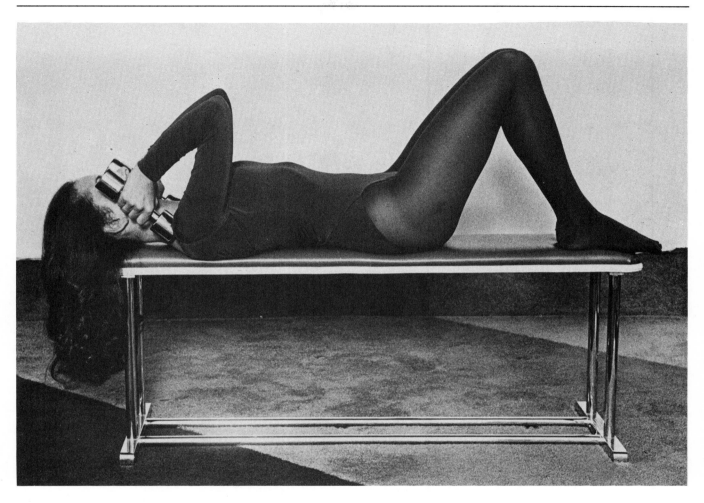

The upper arm extension is the perfect exercise to help eliminate this problem and give your upper arms a youthful look.

Lie flat on your back on a raised bench. Bend your knees with your feet together to prevent a tendency to use the abdominals during this movement. Take a dumbbell in each hand and hold your arms straight up in the air.

Now bend at the elbows and let your hands slowly down to each ear, moving your arms only at the elbows. Press the dumbbells back up with a slow, steady motion.

BREATHING: Exhale as you press dumbbells up; inhale as you let them down.
WEIGHT: 3 pounds, increasing to 5
REPS: 10
SETS: 2, increasing to 3 in the third week

Rest before going to next superset.

SUPERSET 6

PULLOVER WITH DUMBBELL

PURPOSE: To expand the ribcage, improving and increasing the line of your bust.

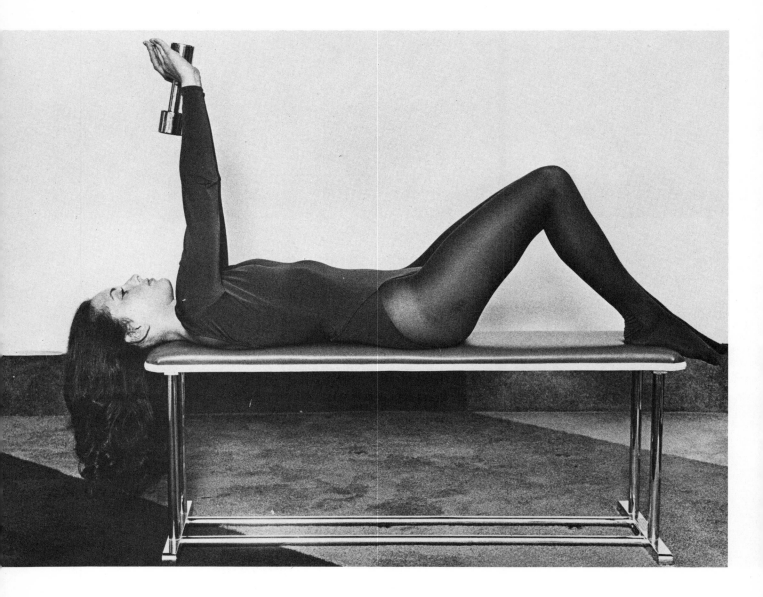

This exercise works the armpit and shoulder portions of the triceps.

Lie flat on a bench with your knees bent. Holding one dumbbell in both hands, raise your arms straight above your chest. Then lower the dumbbell down behind your head, keeping your arms absolutely straight and allowing them to go as low as they will. Pause. Then lift the weight above your chest.

BREATHING: Exhale as you lift the weight; inhale as you lower it behind your head.
WEIGHT: 3 pounds, increasing to 5
REPS: 10, increasing to 20 or 30
SETS: 2, increasing to 3 in the third week

Rest for one minute.

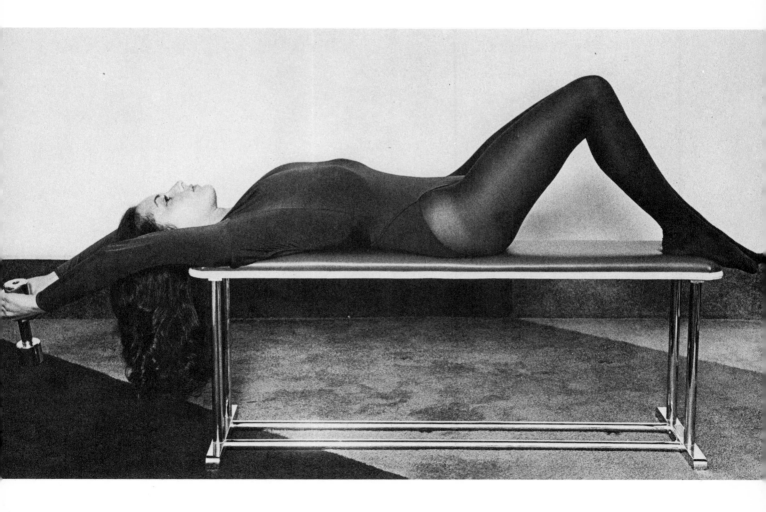

CHEST EXPANDER WITH A WEIGHT

PURPOSE: To firm the bustline.

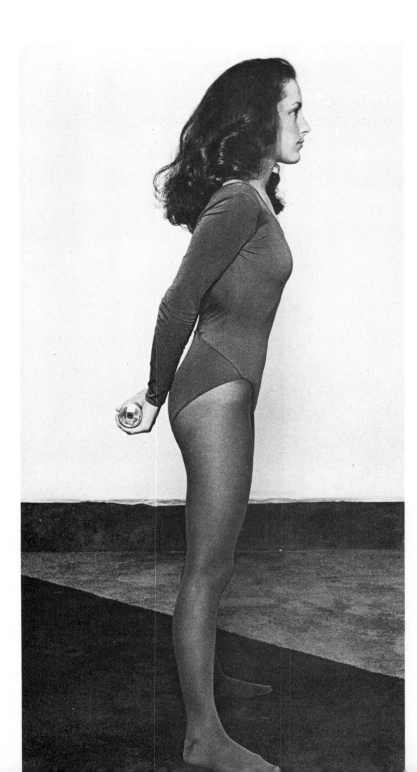

Stand with your feet shoulder width apart. Hold one dumbbell in both hands behind your body, keeping your elbows straight.

Bend forward from the hips, pushing your pelvis down between your thighs without moving your body from the waist to the head, and then reach as far over your head with your arms as you can. Hold this extreme position to a count of 10. This stretches the spine, the buttocks muscles, and the leg biceps. Because of the added weight of the dumbbell, your chest is also expanded.

The number of repetitions or the weight is not as important here as the quality of the movement. You should hold the extreme position as long as possible to get the maximum stretch.

BREATHING: Exhale as you bend forward; inhale as you straighten up.
WEIGHT: 3 pounds, increasing to 5
REPS: 5
SETS: 2, increasing to 3 in the third week

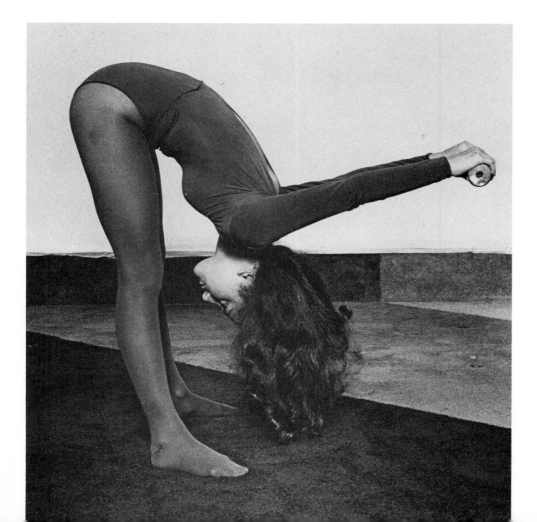

SUPERSET 7

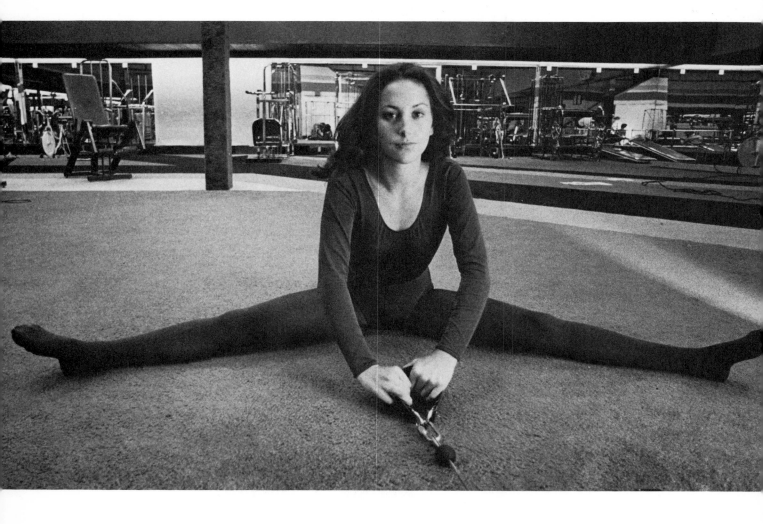

CABLE STRETCH

PURPOSE: To increase flexibility in the hamstrings and lower back.

This stretching exercise is designed to loosen the lower back and hamstrings, areas which are both accident prone.

Sit facing the cable machine and spread your legs as far as possible. Grasp the low pulley collar with both hands and let the

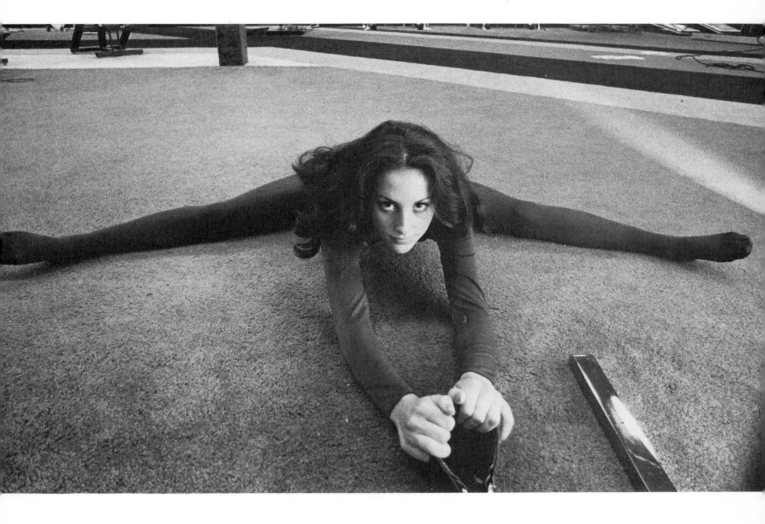

weights slowly pull your arms and torso forward. Pull yourself back to the sitting position; then let yourself go forward again.

Keep your elbows straight and make sure only your pelvis is moving, not the section of your torso above the waist. As a goal, try to work until you can touch your belly-button to the floor. This way the pelvis is being properly stretched.

BREATHING: Exhale as you go forward; inhale as you pull back.
WEIGHT: 20 pounds, increasing to 40
REPS: 10
SETS: 2, increasing to 3 in the third week

STANDING CALF RAISES ON A MACHINE

PURPOSE: To shape and firm the calves.

To get a maximum stretch in your calves, move slowly. Starting with your toes on a high block and your heels on the floor, lift yourself all the way up on your toes, then let your heels all the way down to the floor.

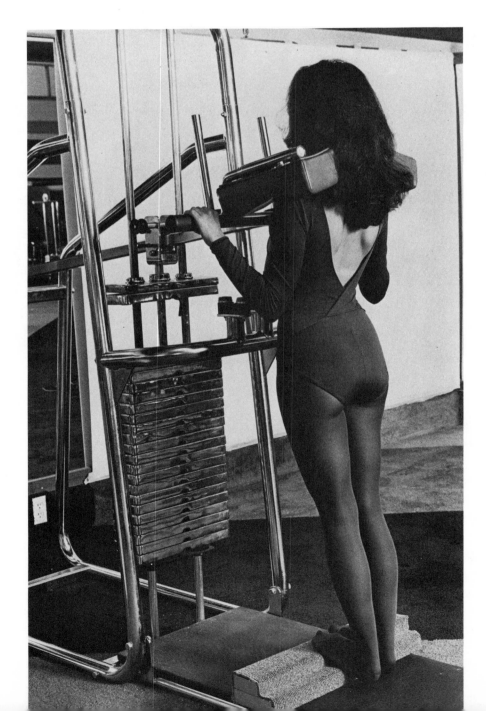

BREATHING: Exhale as you lift up on tiptoe; inhale as you lower
your heels to the floor.
WEIGHT: 50 pounds, increasing to build size
REPS: 20, increasing to reduce size
SETS: 2, increasing to 3 in the third week

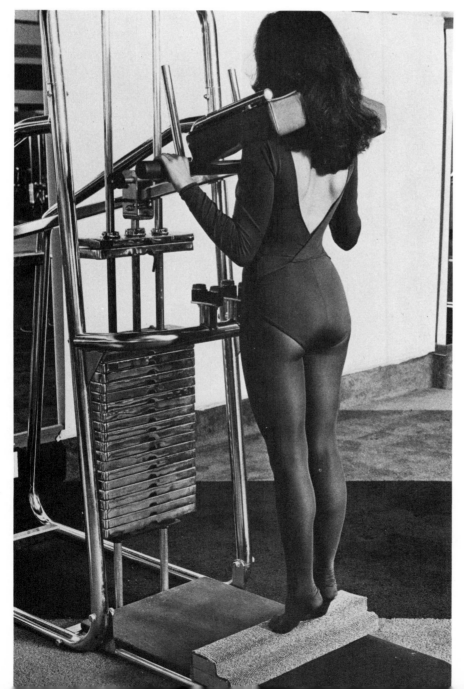

SERIES 4
Exercises for Anytime, Anyplace

THERE IS NO EXCUSE not to exercise. If you cannot go to a gym, you can still go beyond the beginning series and work out at home. When you are traveling, you can exercise in a hotel room or even outdoors. Exercise is too valuable to your life to allow anything to keep you from doing it.

There are a number of advantages to exercising in a gym, and I suggest you go to one if it is at all possible. The atmosphere of a good gym is conducive to working out. There are no phones and no neighbors to drop in during your 45-minute session. The equipment in a gym has been designed to work specific areas of the body and make the exercises that much more beneficial. But not being able to go to a gym is no reason for not continuing with my program. This series provides you with an advanced program which can be done at home or on the road.

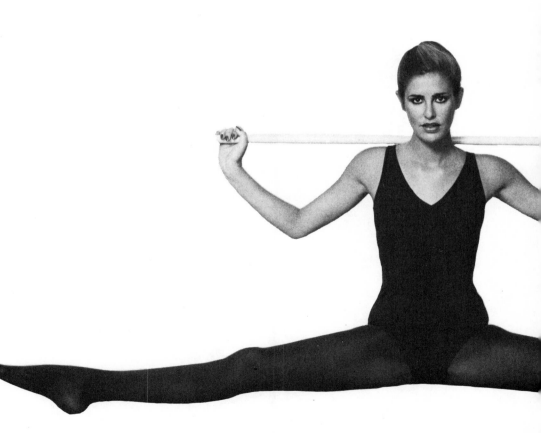

Note: Fewer repetitions with more weight result in building size and mass. More repetitions with less weight result in a decrease of the size of a particular body part.

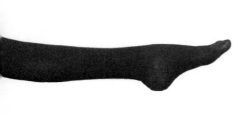

THREE-PART COMBINATION KICK

PURPOSE: To trim the waist, shape the buttocks, smooth the thighs, and flatten the stomach.

This is actually three consecutive exercises done from a single standing position. It works the obliques (the side part of the waist), the buttocks, the entire thigh area, as well as the stomach.

1. Take hold of a chair. This is only for balance and not for assistance. Moving only your leg, kick as high to the front as you can.

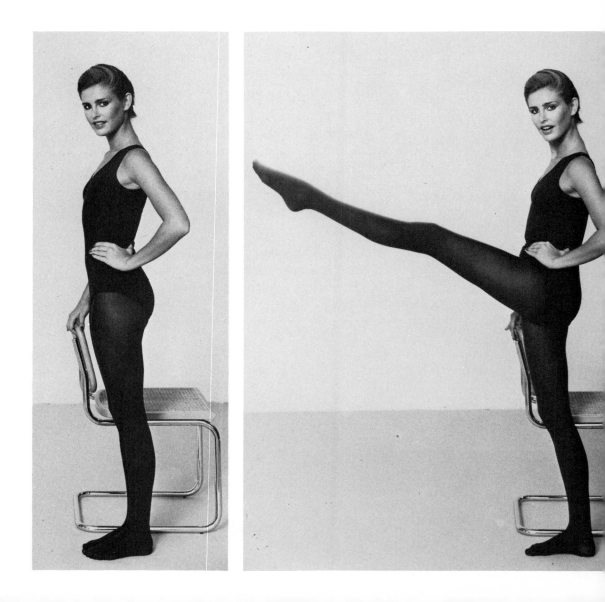

Pause at the highest point. Then let your leg return slowly to the floor, taking full advantage of the negative resistance.

    2. From the same starting position, kick your leg out to the side as far as you can. Pause at the highest point. Then slowly let your leg down. Resist a tendency to lean into the chair.

    3. The final part is a kick to the rear. There is a strong tendency to cheat on this one. Facing the chair back, hold your body upright and your leg straight. Kick as high as you can to the back, pause, lower your leg slowly to the floor.

BREATHING: Exhale as you kick up; inhale as you let your leg down.
REPS: 10 for each of the three parts
SETS: 2, increasing to 3

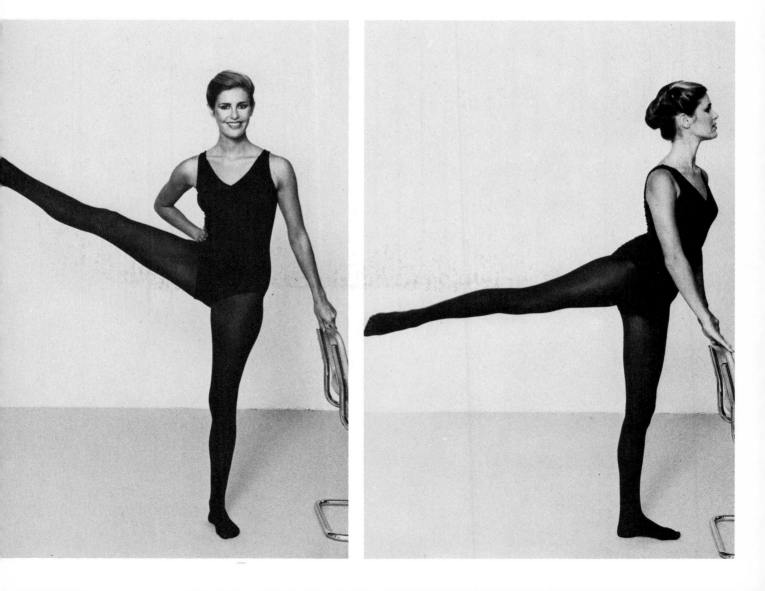

DUMBBELL SQUATS

PURPOSE: To strengthen and firm the thighs.

To begin, take the dumbbells in your hands and stand with your heels on a book or block of wood. Keep your body straight and squat down as low as you can. Do not allow your buttocks to push out when you squat; this will take away from the work of the thighs. Then come back up but do not fully straighten your legs; stop about three-quarters of the way up. Your body should move slowly, smoothly, like a piston.

BREATHING: Exhale as you go down; inhale as you come up.
WEIGHT: 3–5 pounds
REPS: 30
SETS: 2

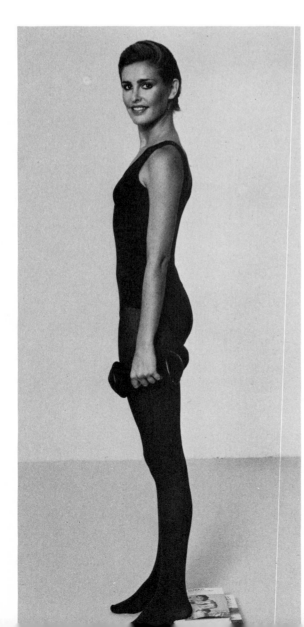

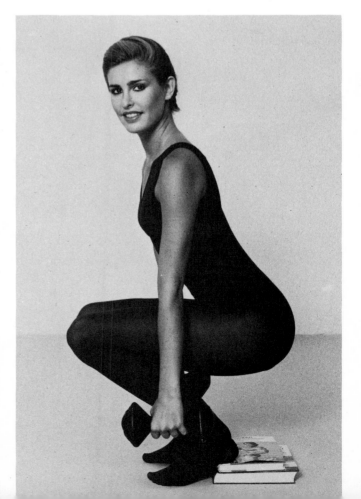

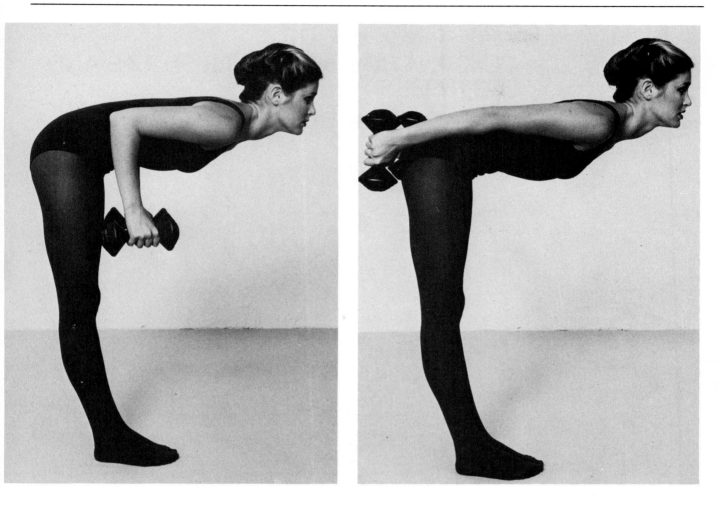

DUMBBELL TRICEPS EXTENSION

PURPOSE: To tighten the muscles at the back of the arm.

Take a dumbbell in each hand. Bend forward, keeping the weights against your thighs. Lift the weights up and back without moving anything except your forearms. If you rotate your forearms or use your upper arms, this will reduce the work of the triceps muscles.

BREATHING: Exhale as you extend your arm; inhale as you let it down.
WEIGHT: 3 pounds
REPS: 10
SETS: 2, increasing to 3

COMBINATION BENT-KNEE SIT-UPS AND LEG RAISES

PURPOSE: To firm and flatten the stomach.

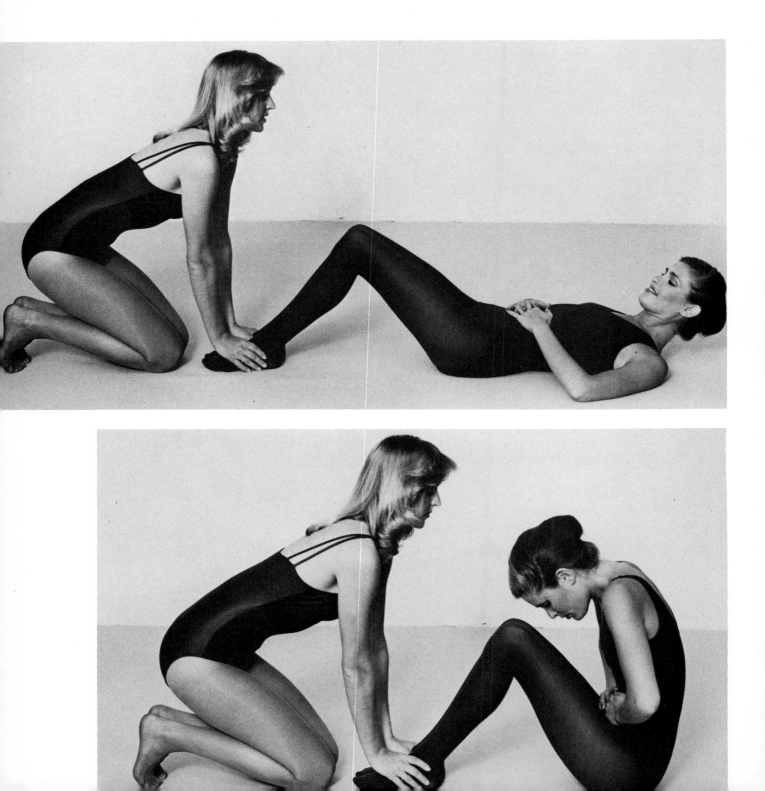

This combination of two exercises tones up the entire stomach—the sit-up for the upper abdominals, the leg raise for the lower abdominals.

Place your feet under a heavy piece of furniture, such as a bed, with your legs bent at a 45-degree angle (to prevent the back from doing any of the work). Or enlist the aid of a friend. Starting with your back on the floor, pull yourself up and then let yourself back down. You should do these movements as fast as you can, establishing a smooth definite rhythm. If this exercise irritates your tailbone, sit on a folded towel.

Without resting, while still on your back, place your hands, palm down, under your buttocks and extend your legs out straight. Tuck your chin slightly and pull your legs as far as you can into your chest area. Thrust them back into the straight position and immediately bring them into the chest.

BREATHING: Exhale as you sit up; inhale as you return to floor.
Exhale as you lift your legs; inhale as you lower them.
REPS: 20 for each exercise, increasing to 50
SETS: 2 for each exercise, increasing to 3

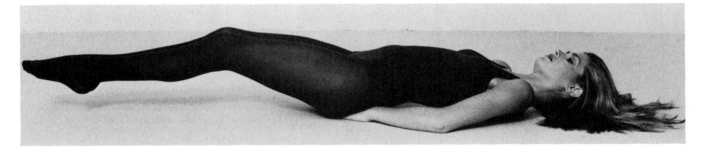

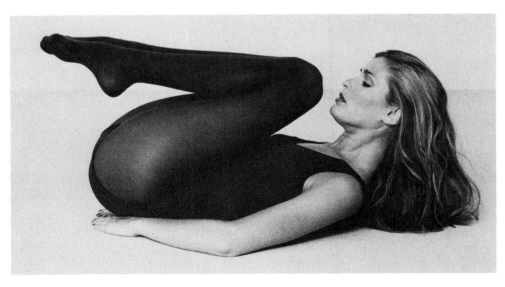

SITTING TWISTS

PURPOSE: To slenderize the waist.

Sit on the floor with your back straight and your legs spread as wide as you can without straining. Place a broomstick across your shoulders and grip the ends firmly. Swing to the right, trying to bring your left arm at least parallel to your right leg. Swing back to the left, bringing your right arm parallel with your left leg. Keep your back straight and your legs flat on the floor and concentrate the action in your waist.

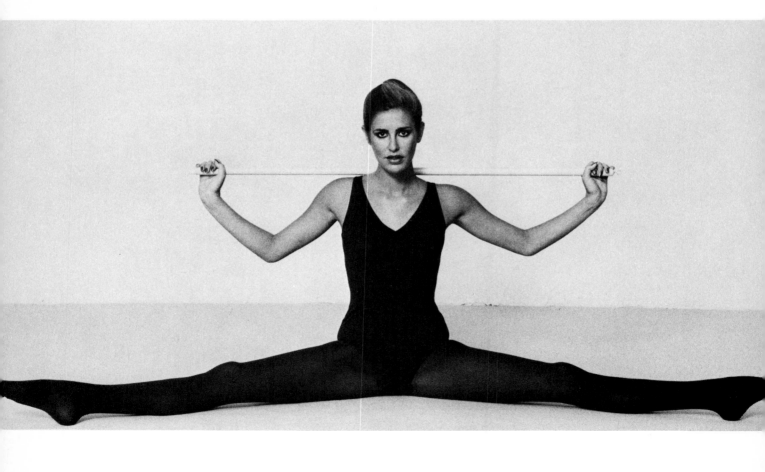

BREATHING: Breathe with an easy rhythm—in to the left; out to the
right.
REPS: In the beginning, I recommend 15 fast repetitions to
each side, which is a total of 30. Increase, depending
on need, to at least 50.
SETS: 2

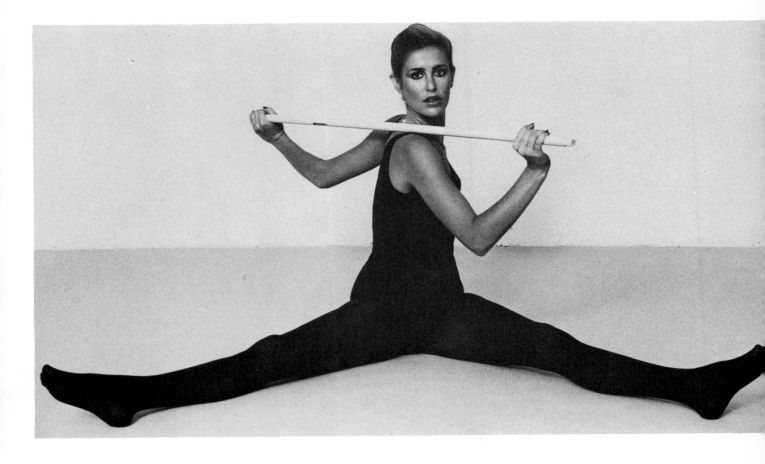

CALF RAISES WITH DUMBBELL

PURPOSE: To tone, build, and smooth the calves.

You should be familiar with the basic movements of this exercise. But as a variation, add two alternate foot positions and work with a single dumbbell. Always hold the weight on the side of the calf you are exercising:

1. Stand with your toes pointed out and your heels pointed in.
2. Stand with your heels pointed out and your toes pointed in.

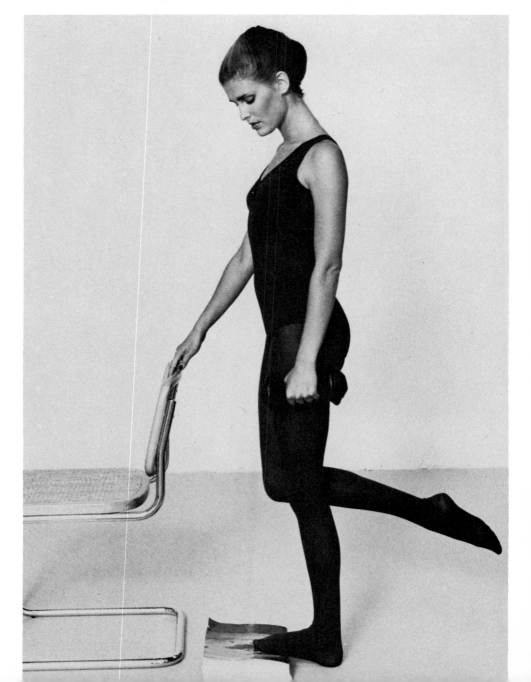

You will immediately feel the difference this makes to the calf muscle. Keep the movements slow and really stretch your calves.

BREATHING: Exhale as you go up on tiptoe; inhale as you lower your heel to the floor.
WEIGHT: 3–5 pounds
REPS: 10, increasing to 20
SETS: 2, increasing to 3

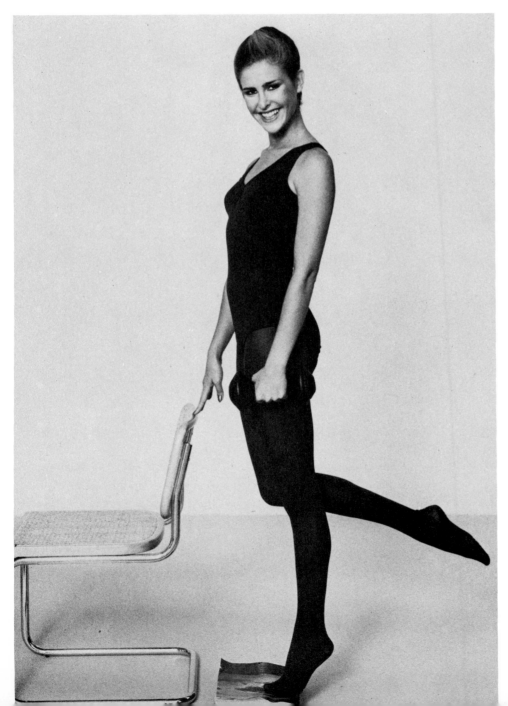

CHAIR OR COUNTER PUSH-UPS

PURPOSE: To develop the pectoral muscles and increase the bustline.

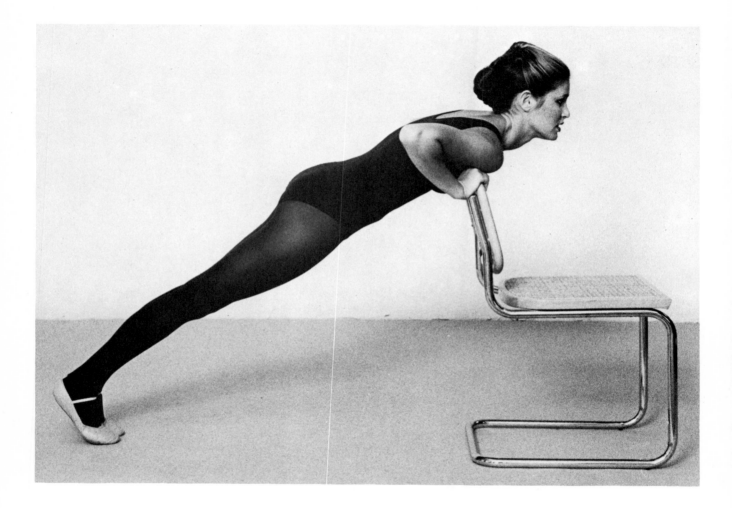

You need a chair, counter, or table for this exercise.

Stand with your feet spaced 6 or 8 inches apart and your toes about 3 feet from the chair back (later you can increase this distance to add more resistance). Your hands should be approximately 18 inches apart on the chair back, with the elbows pointing out (keeping the elbows turned out concentrates the work on the pectoral area and not in the backs of the arms). Let yourself down slowly until you barely touch the edge of the chair back; then push back to the beginning

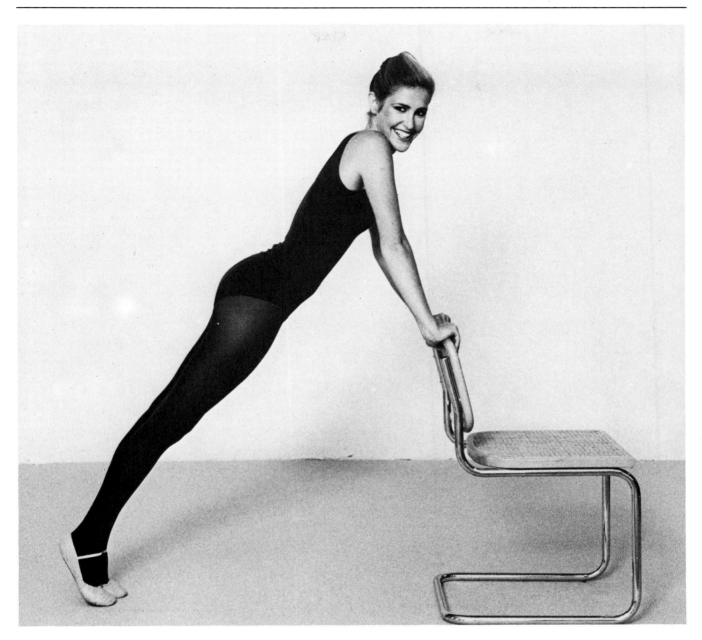

position. When this becomes easy with the suggested number of reps, increase the distance between your toes and the chair.

BREATHING: Exhale as you push up from the counter; inhale as you lower your body.

REPS: 15

SETS: 2, increasing to 3

THE COMPLETE BACKLIFT

PURPOSE: To strengthen and tone the lower back and buttocks.

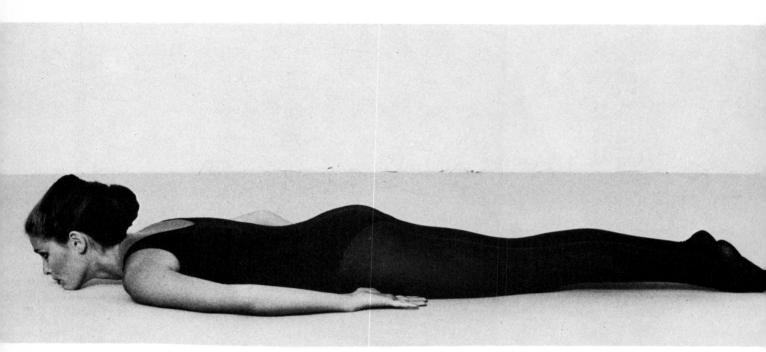

Many women have a weak lower back, which causes problems and often affects their posture. This modification of a popular yoga exercise will help strengthen the muscles in that neglected area.

Lie on your stomach, holding your legs together and your arms at your sides. Tuck your chin slightly.

Breathe deeply before you begin, expanding your lungs. Arch up with your neck and then your back, as you see in the photograph. Let yourself back to the floor slowly. Repeat. Note: This exercise is not

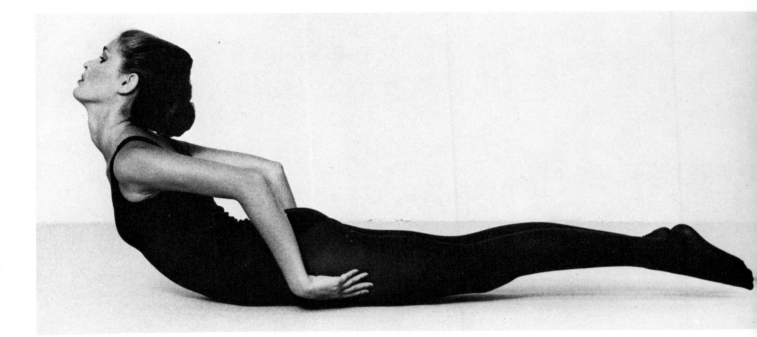

to be done rigidly. Do not strain. Lift yourself up only as much as you can. You will improve as you strengthen your lower back muscles.

BREATHING: Exhale as you lift your body; inhale as you return to the floor.
REPS: 10
SETS: 2

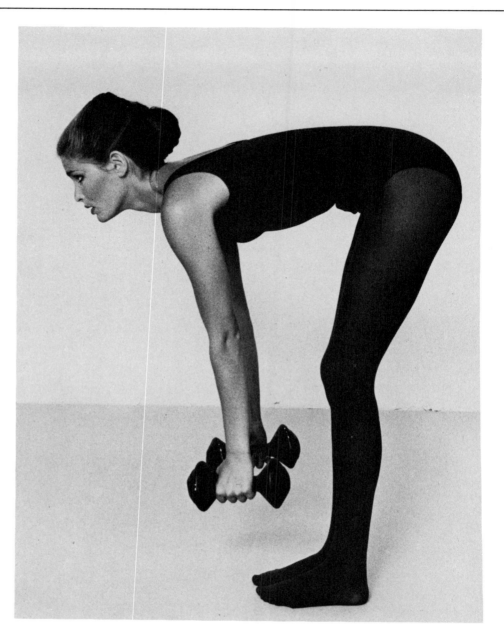

DUMBBELL ROWING

PURPOSE: To straighten the center of the lower back and the entire upper back.

Hold a dumbbell in each hand and bend forward until your upper body is parallel to the floor. Keep your knees slightly bent and your palms facing each other. Slowly pull the weights up, to touch the

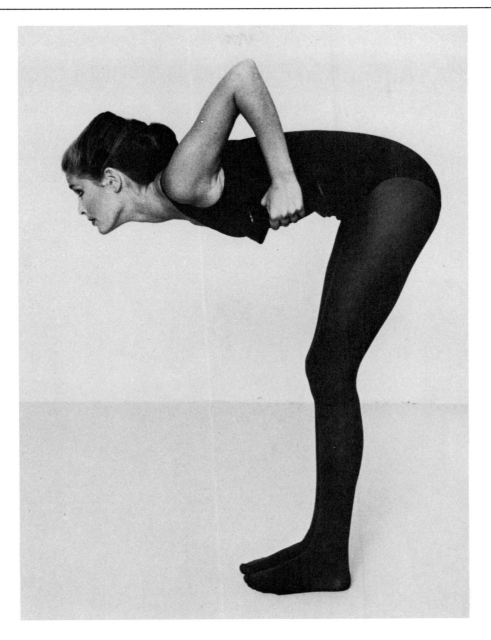

sides of your waist. Let them down slowly to get the full benefit of negative resistance.

BREATHING: Exhale as you pull up; inhale as you lower the weights.
WEIGHT: 3–5 pounds
REPS: 10
SETS: 2, increasing to 3

ALTERNATE FRONT DUMBBELL RAISES

PURPOSE: To strengthen, tone, and smooth the shoulders.

Take a dumbbell in each hand and stand with your back straight and your feet approximately 10 inches apart. Begin with your arms straight and your palms facing your thighs.

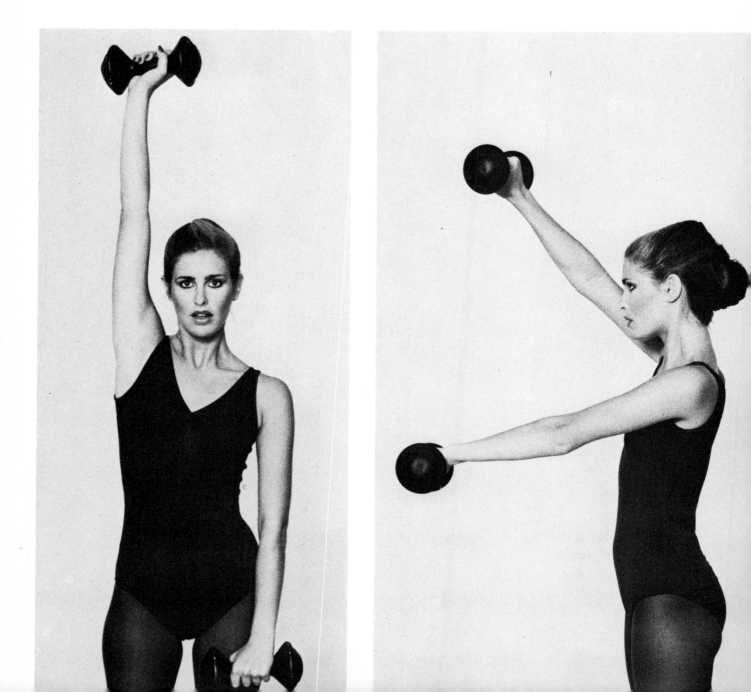

Lift your right arm over your head. As you are lowering your right arm, raise your left arm over your head. The movement should be simultaneous, the dumbbells passing at shoulder height. Do not pause or allow your arms to rotate.

BREATHING: Rhythmical
WEIGHT: 3–5 pounds
REPS: 10 with each arm
SETS: 2, increasing to 3

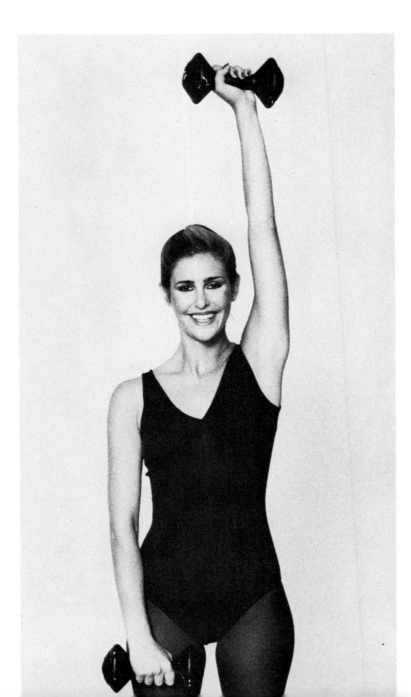

DUMBBELL CURLS

PURPOSE: To strengthen the biceps.

This exercise is found in Series 1 on page 73.
BREATHING: Exhale as you lift; inhale as you lower weight.
WEIGHT: 3–5 pounds
REPS: 10
SETS: 2, increasing to 3

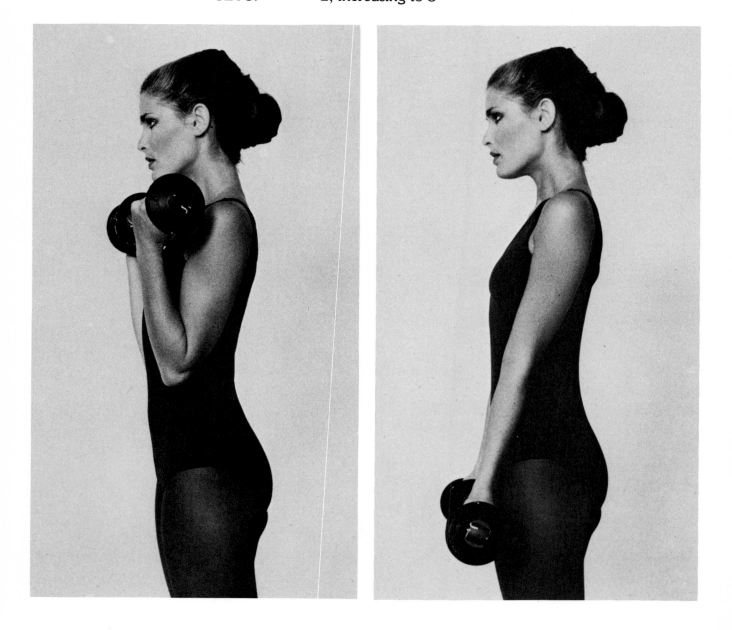

Problem Areas

No woman's body is the same as another's. One woman will need more work on her waist, another will want to improve her shoulders, a third has endless trouble with her thighs. For this reason, I have included two photographs for easy reference to the various exercises that work specific parts or areas of the body.

Remember, while you are working on a specific area, you should not neglect the rest of your body. Simply cut back on the number of sets in your best areas and add more sets to exercises for your problem areas.

PECTORALS

Push-ups
from the Knees,
page 66
Bench Press, page 85
Dumbbell Flys, page 112
Chair or Counter Push-ups,
page 138

ABDOMINALS

Elevated Leg
Crunches,
page 60
Bent-Knee Sit-ups, page 88
Two-Part Leg Raises,
page 98
Three-Part Combination
Kick, page 128
Combination Sit-ups/Leg
Raises, page 132

OUTER THIGH

Leg Lift, page 54
Outer Thigh Cable Pulls,
page 76
Kneeling Cable Pulls,
page 102

FRONTAL THIGH

Leg Press on a Machine,
page 80
Leg Extensions, page 82
Parallel Squats, page 106

LOWER FRONTAL THIGH

Leg Extensions, page 82

WAIST

Three-Part Combination
Kick, page 128
Sitting Twists, page 134
Waist Slimmer, page 62
Twists with a Broomstick,
page 71
Twists on a Machine,
page 92
Side Bends with a Cable,
page 100
Three-Way Stretch, pages
51 and 52

INNER THIGH

Scissor Leg Lift, page 56
Inner Thigh Cable Pulls,
page 78
Sitting Cable Pulls, page
104
Cable Stretch, page 122
Three-Way Stretch, pages
51 and 52

SHOULDERS

Front Press with Barbell,
page 86
Side Laterals with
Dumbbells, pages 72 and
114
Alternate Front Dumbbell
Raises, page 144
Warm-Ups, page 48

BICEPS

Dumbbell Curls, pages 73
and 146
Reverse Curls, page 94

RIBCAGE

Chest Expander with a
Weight, page 120
Pullover with Dumbbell,
page 118

FOREARMS

Reverse Curls, page 94

CALVES

Calf Raises, page 68
Standing Calf Raises on a
Machine, pages 84 and 124
Calf Raises with Dumbbell,
page 136

UPPER BACK

Pull-ups Between Chairs,
page 70
Narrow Grip Pulldown,
page 110
Dumbbell Rowing, page
142
Beginning Stretches, pages
49 and 50

TRICEPS

Triceps Push-up, page 64
Upper Arm Extensions,
page 116
Dumbbell Triceps
Extension, page 131

LOWER BACK

Cable Stretch, page 122
The Complete Backlift,
page 140
Dumbbell Rowing, page
142
Warm-Ups, page 48

BUTTOCKS

Rear Leg Lift, page 58
Parallel Squats, page 106
Three-Part Combination
Kick, page 128
Dumbbell Squats, page 130

LEG BICEPS

Leg Curls on a Machine,
page 108
Leg Press on a Machine,
page 80
Dumbbell Squats, page 130
Parallel Squats, page 106
Beginning Stretches, pages
49 and 50

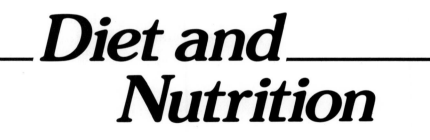

Diet and Nutrition

A Commonsense Approach to Good Eating

Everyone is on a diet. The problem is that many times our diet does not coincide with our goals. If you want to lose fat, you must adjust your diet accordingly. Ordinarily this will not mean drastic changes, only sensible adjustments.

American women are forever dieting. Diets and diet aids are big business. In a single year, Americans spend more than ten billion dollars on diet aids. I am not criticizing the impulse behind dieting, but there is a better, healthier way to trim inches from your waist, thighs, buttocks, or any other part of your body. Fad diets, crash weight-loss programs, and chemical dietary aids fail to work because they are not compatible with continuous good health. To do it right, you must change your eating habits—the way you eat, how much you eat, and what you eat—and when you find the diet that best suits you, then stick with it.

I cannot promise that you will lose 20 pounds in 20 days; instead, the losses you will experience through exercise and a sensible diet will be gradual, natural, easy for your system to accept, and effortless for you to maintain.

Look at it this way: Your excess fat has accumulated over a long period. You tolerated it for that length of time, so why are you in such a hurry to get rid of it? You have plenty of time to lose it, especially when you consider that this loss is going to be permanent.

In any really successful diet, there are no magical formulas. Substituting good eating habits for the poor ones that took a lifetime to acquire is the biggest battle. The basic principle for cutting down your body to the size you want it to be is to *eat fewer calories than you burn.* Therefore, it stands to reason that if you do not increase your present calorie intake and add 3 hours of vigorous exercise to your regimen of weekly activity, you will begin to lose both inches and pounds. This can be further accelerated by reducing the number of calories you take in.

No diet should eliminate any essential nutrient. Every body, even an obese body, needs a balance of proteins, carbohydrates, and fats, plus all the vitamins and minerals. We know the American diet contains far too much fat, far too many empty calories from carbohydrates. This does not mean you should cut out fats and carbohydrates completely. But you can reduce the amount of fat and select carbohydrates of a better quality. For most of you, the solution is to substitute fish and chicken (with the skin removed) for red meat, to use fat-free or low-fat dairy products, to eat plenty of fresh vegetables (raw when possible), and to cut out desserts and other foods made with sugar, eating fresh fruit in their place.

1. There is only one way to reduce. You must put into your body less than the amount required to maintain it in its overweight state. This can be accomplished best through a combination of doing more exercise and eating less high-carbohydrate food.

2. You must not underestimate the value of exercise during the time you are trying to improve your eating habits. Exercise alleviates hunger, improves your self-image, and helps build optimism about the future. Dieting without exercise can leave you with loose sagging skin and slack muscles and make you look and feel worse than you did before you began your diet.

3. If you do not increase your food intake, regular exercise as I am prescribing it will make you lose pounds, trim off inches, and firm up.

4. Exercise is excellent for digestion. People who exercise regularly are less prone to constipation and kidney stones. Exercise normalizes your eating habits by combating stress and helping to eliminate the compulsive eating habits so many women seem to have.

Diet and Exercise to Avoid Sagging Skin and Slack Muscles

I believe proper nutrition is at least 50 percent of physical fitness. Therefore, in order to cultivate the good eating habits necessary to maintain a perfect body, you should know the essentials of nutrition. I have outlined them briefly. If you have a specific problem, I suggest you consult a nutritionist.

Some Basics of Nutrition

PROTEIN. Protein is responsible for the growth, maintenance, and repair of muscle tissue. Without sufficient high-grade protein, the body actually begins to deteriorate. The chief functions of proteins are to provide nitrogen and amino acids for the body proteins (skin tissue, organs, muscles, brain, hair, etc.) and to stimulate the production of hormones that affect cell activity, antibodies to fight infection and disease, and enzymes to control the chemical reactions in the body.

Proteins fall into two classifications: complete proteins, which contain all the essential amino acids; and incomplete proteins, which lack one or more of the amino acids. Eggs, lean meat, fish, chicken, and yogurt are examples of complete proteins. Incomplete proteins are rice, beans, lentils, and wheat germ. Obviously, the best sources of protein are the complete proteins; however, by combining two incomplete proteins, such as rice and beans, a complete protein can be formed. Incomplete proteins can also be utilized when served with a complete protein: fish and rice, for example.

CARBOHYDRATES. Carbohydrates are necessary in your diet as a source of energy, or fuel as I like to call it. They provide vital glucose for the various brain functions, digest protein, and make protein enzymes utilizable. Without carbohydrates, your body would burn protein for energy and prevent it from serving its main functions—building, repair, and maintenance.

The best sources of carbohydrates are vegetables, fruits, whole grain breads, and dairy products. Those to avoid are sugar, sugar products, and highly refined flours.

FATS. Fats heat and lubricate the body, insulate and protect important organs, provide essential fatty acids, and give you a base for carrying Vitamins A, D, and E. Fats should never be eliminated totally from your diet. Some fats, however, are preferable to others. Saturated fats—animal fats, lard, and shortening—are the least desirable. Polyunsaturated fats—safflower oil and corn oil are good examples—are excellent sources of the kind of fats your body really needs.

VITAMINS AND MINERALS. I am not a fanatic about vitamins and minerals. I always try to eat the highest quality fresh foods I can get, but I can never be sure of their nutritional value. So I take vitamins as insurance. For years, I have been using supplements conveniently packaged into daily dosages. Each pack supplies my body with the minimum daily requirement of all the necessary vitamins and all but the most esoteric minerals. (Note that I take them as a *supplement* and never as a *substitute* for wholesome food.) Because I rarely operate at a minimum, I recognize that there are times when I will require additional supplements. If I am under the additional pressure of seminars or public appearances, I increase the number of vitamin packs to two or three and sometimes four a day.

Unless you are a chemist and qualified to combine vitamins and minerals in their correct proportions, I suggest you adopt a similar supplement program. In making your selection, read the label carefully. Be certain the formula contains all the vitamins and minerals listed below.

Vitamin A promotes good vision, helps prevent infection, and maintains the tissues covering the body surfaces—both inner surfaces (linings of the mouth, throat, lungs, nostrils, intestinal tract) and outer surfaces (skin). It also protects the tissues that line the interiors of the glands and is essential to bone development, appetite, and digestion.

B-complex vitamins include B_1, B_2, B_3, B_6, folic acid, PABA, pantothenic acid, biotin, B_{12}, choline, and inositol. The B-complex vitamins work in unison to protect the body against fatigue, tension, depression, and other nervous disorders. They help digestion; feed the brain, skin, blood, and *eyes*; and are vital in the production of essential enzymes for the synthesis of amino acids.

Vitamin C benefits the nervous system, circulatory system, muscles, and all connective tissues. It is needed for normal blood clotting and helps wounds heal. Vitamin C is not stored in the body, so constant replenishment is necessary.

Vitamin D helps to absorb and utilize the minerals calcium and phosphorous, both of which are important in building and maintaining strong bones and teeth.

Vitamin E is an antioxidant, which means it acts to prevent certain fatty acids and such vitamins as A and D from combining with oxygen and being destroyed. This, in turn, reduces the body's need for oxygen and, therefore, makes vitamin E valuable to anyone engaging in vigorous exercise.

I recommend you take vitamins three times a day, always with a meal.

If you take them only once a day, take them at breakfast. Never take them on an empty stomach. They need the proteins and enzymes from foods to be fully effective. Then, too, on an empty stomach, they can cause indigestion.

MINERALS. Your body uses a large number of minerals in its functions, only a few of which you need to consider in choosing your supplements.

Calcium is needed more abundantly than any other mineral. It is necessary for strong teeth and bones, normal blood clotting, and regulating the activities of both the muscles and nerves. Calcium has been called nature's tranquilizer: It fights tension, irritability, and insomnia.

Magnesium works with calcium to build bones, and with phosphorous and the enzymes to maintain muscle and nerve equilibrium.

Iron is an important ingredient in hemoglobin, the part of the blood responsible for transporting oxygen to the cells. Due to hormonal development, menstruation, and menopause, women need iron in greater quantities than men.

Copper is vital to healthy hair and skin. A deficiency can cause anemia.

Zinc promotes good circulation (working here in conjunction with copper), assists in healing processes, and helps keep the skin strong and supple.

Phosphorous works as a catalyst in changing the basic food elements into energy. It is essential to strong bones and healthy teeth.

Iodine helps regulate the thyroid gland and therefore has a direct affect on energy in the body.

Two Commonsense Diets for Losing Weight During Resistance Training

TO LOSE A LITTLE. If you need to lose only an inch here and there or a few pounds, your problem is relatively simple. You can take care of it by restricting the number of calories you consume. To do this, buy a calorie counter in a drugstore or health-food store to determine the number of calories in the food you consume in a typical day. If the number is 1,500, then you might cut back to 1,350. If it is 1,000, try 850 or 900. Just remember that the foods to cut back are carbohydrates and saturated fats. Never reduce your protein intake. However, you may find that you can easily substitute better quality proteins for the ones you now consume: Fish and skinless chicken are more desirable than beef or pork; low fat dairy products are better than ordinary dairy products. Stay on this diet for a couple of weeks, measuring and weighing yourself twice a week, at the same time each day. If you find you are not making progress, cut back a little more. Keep exercising according to the schedule I've outlined in this book and take your vitamin and mineral supplements. Once you have reached your desired size/weight goal, you can adjust your intake just enough to maintain it.

TO LOSE MORE. If you need to lose more than a few inches and pounds, the best approach is a low-carbohydrate diet. Limit yourself to from 30 to 60 grams of carbohydrates per day, but don't cut them out altogether. In some ways, this diet is less complicated than the first diet because you don't have to worry about counting the calories of everything you eat; you count only the grams of carbohydrates. This diet will not leave you feeling hungry. High-carbohydrate foods act to stimulate the appetite; proteins satisfy the appetite. When you eat fewer carbohydrates, your body utilizes the excess fat it has stored for energy. Stay away from any foods with sugar or refined flour in them. Eat fish, meat, fowl, cheese, fresh vegetables, and low-carbohydrate fruit, such as strawberries and cantaloupe. Check the list on the following page for the carbohydrate gram count of the more popular foods.

Note: It is important in this and any diet to eat at least three small meals a day. Breakfast is important and should never be skipped. With it, you should take your vitamin and mineral supplements.

	Portion	Calories	Grams of Carbohy- drates
Beverages			
Beer	8 oz	101	10.8
Coffee	8 oz	2	.8
Cola drink	8 oz	88	22
Dry wine	8 oz	204	9.6
Martini	3½ oz	140	.3
Skim milk	8 oz	89	13
Whole milk	8 oz	159	12
Bread & Cereals			
Bran flakes 40%	1 cup (40 gm)	143	30.8
Corn flakes	1 cup (25 gm)	98	21
Oatmeal, cooked	1 cup (236 gm)	130	23
Rye	1 slice (23 gm)	56	12
Whole wheat	1 slice (23 gm)	55	11
Condiments & Sauces			
Cider vinegar	1 tb (15 gm)	3	.9
French dressing	1 tb (15 gm)	62	2.6
Hollandaise	1 tb (21 gm)	48	1.6
Italian dressing	1 tb (15 gm)	83	1.0
Mayonnaise	1 tb (14 gm)	101	.3
Mustard	1 tb (12 gm)	11	.5
Soy sauce	1 tb (15 gm)	8	1.5
Tomato catsup	1 tb (17 gm)	19	4.3
Cream			
Half-&-Half	1 tb (15 gm)	20	.7
Whipping	1 cup (8 oz)	860	7.4
Dairy Products			
Cheddar cheese	1 oz	112	.6
Cottage cheese	1 cup (8 oz)	235	6.5
Cream cheese	1 tb (14 gm)	53	.3
Gruyere cheese	1 oz	115	.5
Swiss cheese	1 oz	99	.5
Desserts			
Apple pie	1 piece (135 gm)	346	50
Brownies	1 slice (50 gm)	243	25
Cake doughnuts	1 med	33	17
Chocolate chip cookies	1 med (9 gm)	46	5.3

	Portion	Calories	Grams of Carbohy-drates
Devils food cake, no icing	1 slice (45 gm)	165	23.4
Ice cream, all flavors	1 cup	389	39
Peanut cookie	1 large (14 gm)	66	9
Pumpkin pie	1 piece (130 gm)	274	30
Sugar	1 tb (12 gm)	46	12

Eggs

	Portion	Calories	Grams of Carbohy-drates
Boiled, poached or raw	1 med	79	.4
Fried	1 med	108	.4

Fats & Oils

	Portion	Calories	Grams of Carbohy-drates
Butter	1 tb (14 gm)	100	.1
Safflower oil	1 tb (14 gm)	124	0

Fish & Sea Foods

	Portion	Calories	Grams of Carbohy-drates
Bluefish, baked or broiled	1 lb	720	0
Cod, broiled	1 lb	740	0
Crabmeat	1 lb	398	2.3
Lobster, steamed	1 med (200 gm)	179	.6
Oysters, raw	1 cup (240 gm)	152	15.4
Salmon, broiled	1 lb	824	0

Fruits & Juices

	Portion	Calories	Grams of Carbohy-drates
Apple	1 med (130 gm)	76	17
Avocado	1 large (216 gm)	361	12
Banana	1 med (150 gm)	128	30
Blueberries	1 cup (140 gm)	87	19
Cantaloupe	¼ (100 gm)	30	7.5
Dried dates	1 med (10 gm)	27	6.3
Dried figs	1 med (38 gm)	30	6.8
Grapefruit	1 med (260 gm)	108	25
Lemon juice	1 tb (15 gm)	4	1.2
Ripe olives	1 large (7 gm)	13	.2
Papaya	1 large (400 gm)	156	40
Peach	1 med (114 gm)	43	10
Pear	1 med (182 gm)	111	27.8
Raisins	1 cup (160 gm)	462	111
Raspberries	1 cup (133 gm)	76	16
Strawberries	1 cup (149 gm)	55	11

	Portion	Calories	Grams of Carbohydrates
Grains			
Brown rice, raw	1 cup (190 gm)	744	161
Wheat bran	1 oz (29 gm)	62	17.9
Wheat germ	1 tb (6 gm)	24	2.7
White rice, raw	1 cup (191 gm)	675	154
Meat, Poultry & Game			
Beef round steak, lean	1 lb (435 gm)	856	0
Chicken, broiled no skin	(453 gm)	616	0
Ham	1 lb (435 gm)	1309	0
Hamburger, reg. cooked	4 oz (86 gm)	188	0
Lamb leg, roasted	(453 gm)	1264	0
Pork roast	1 lb (435 gm)	1690	0
Sirloin, T-bone, porterhouse	1 lb (435 gm)	1848	0
Turkey, white meat	1 lb (435 gm)	797	0
Nuts			
Almonds, dried	1 cup (140 gm)	765	26
Cashews, unsalted	1 cup (100 gm)	569	26
Peanut butter	1 tb (15 gm)	88	2.8
Roasted peanuts	1 cup (240 gm)	1418	45
Sesame seeds	1 cup (230 gm)	1339	41
Vegetables			
Artichoke	1 small (100 gm)	44	9.9
Asparagus	1 spear (16 gm)	3.2	0.6
Baked potato	1 med (100 gm)	93	21.1
Beansprouts	1 cup (50 gm)	18	3.3
Broccoli	1 cup (150 gm)	39	6.8
Carrot, raw	1 large (100 gm)	42	9.7
Cauliflower, raw	1 cup (100 gm)	27	5.2
Celery stalk, raw	1 large (50 gm)	8	2
Corn, whole kernel	1 cup (200 gm)	132	31.4
Cucumber, raw	½ med (50 gm)	8	1.7
Green beans, cooked	1 cup (125 gm)	31	8.9
Green onions	1 bulb (8 gm)	4	0.8
Green pepper	1 large (100 gm)	22	4.8
Iceberg lettuce	3½ oz (100 gm)	13	2.9
Lima beans, cooked	1 cup (195 gm)	265	49.0
Spinach, steamed	1 cup (100 gm)	23	3.6
Tomato, raw	1 med (150 gm)	33	7.1

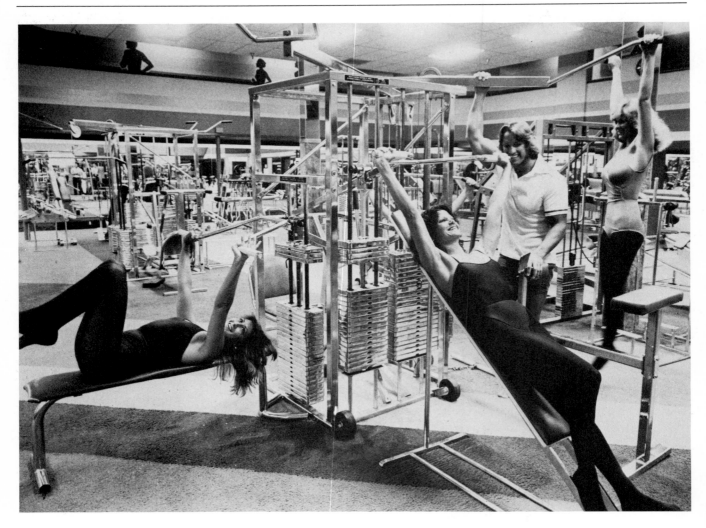

Beyond This Book

When you have completed the first three or four months of exercises, you should know your body well enough to be able to devise your own maintenance program. Remember always to include exercises for every area of your body. Do not neglect a certain area just because it never causes you problems. Balance is the key to a really vital and healthy body. And staying fit and beautiful is something you should want to work on for the rest of your life. Look at it as being as essential to your total well-being as eating. You must eat for the rest of your life in order to stay alive; and you should stay in shape in order to get the most out of your life.

Arnold